MW00997904

About the Authors

Todd A. Smitherman, PhD, FAHS, is Associate Professor of Psychology and Director of the Center for Behavioral Medicine at the University of Mississippi. He has published over 50 peer-reviewed journal articles and numerous book chapters, most pertaining to psychiatric comorbidities and other behavioral issues in headache disorders. His research has been supported by the Migraine Research Foundation, the American Headache Society, the University of Mississippi, and Merck Pharmaceuticals. Dr. Smitherman serves as associate editor for *Headache: The Journal of Head and Face Pain*, is a fellow of the American Headache Society and chair of its Behavioral Issues Section, and has served as a consultant for the Common Data Elements Working Group for Headache Clinical Trials (National Institute of Neurological Disorders and Stroke).

Donald B. Penzien, PhD, FAHS, is widely recognized for his expertise and contributions in headache research methodologies and development of cost-efficient behavioral interventions for headache (i.e., limited-therapist-contact therapies). He presently serves as Professor of Anesthesiology at the Wake Forest School of Medicine. In 1986, he founded the Head Pain Center at University of Mississippi Medical Center, where he served as Director and Professor of Psychiatry until 2014. He is a fellow of the American Headache Society and the Society of Behavioral Medicine. He has published extensively in behavioral medicine, with over 150 research articles, book chapters, and monographs to his credit. His work has been supported by grants from the National Institutes of Health, Department of Defense, and other funding agencies. He is associate editor for *Headache: The Journal of Head and Face Pain,* has served on editorial boards of other scientific journals, and has actively served numerous professional organizations. Key appointments have included chair of the Nonpharmacologic Therapies Review Group for the Headache Treatment Guidelines Project (Agency for Healthcare Research and Quality), Board of Directors as well as chair of the Behavioral Clinical Trials Guidelines Workgroup (American Headache Society), member of the US Headache Treatment Guidelines Consortium (American Academy of Neurology), and member of the Common Data Elements Working Group for Headache Clinical Trials (National Institute of Neurological Disorders and Stroke).

Jeanetta C. Rains, PhD, FAHS, is Clinical Director of the Center for Sleep Evaluation at Elliot Hospital in Manchester, New Hampshire. She is a fellow of the American Board of Sleep Medicine, the American Academy of Sleep Medicine, and the American Headache Society. She is a leading authority in the field of headache and sleep medicine, having worked in this area since 1991. She has authored more than 90 scientific publications. She is associate editor for *Headache: The Journal of Head and Face Pain* and serves on the editorial board for the *Journal of Applied Psychophysiology and Biofeedback.* Her research has been supported by the American Headache Society and Merck Pharmaceuticals, and she has served as a consultant for research supported by the Migraine Research Foundation and American Headache Foundation.

Robert A. Nicholson, PhD, FAHS, is Director of Research for Mercy Health System and Director of Behavioral Medicine at Mercy Health Research and Mercy Clinic Headache Center. He earned his doctorate in clinical psychology (specializing in behavioral medicine) at Virginia Commonwealth University and completed a predoctoral internship and postdoctoral research fellowship at Brown University Medical School. His research and clinical focus is on the use of maximally effective patient communication strategies for prevention and management of migraine and integrating patient reports into optimal migraine treatment design. He has received grants from the National Institute of Neurological Disorders and Stroke, the National Cancer Institute, the National Headache Foundation, Saint Louis University, and the private sector to support his research. Dr. Nicholson has published extensively and made numerous presentations at scientific and professional conferences.

Timothy T. Houle, PhD, is Associate Professor of Anesthesiology at Wake Forest School of Medicine. He has published over 80 peer-reviewed journal articles and numerous book chapters principally addressing chronic pain and the triggers of headache, and much of his research has focused on the prediction of headache attacks in the individual. His work has been funded by the National Institute of Neurological Disorders and Stroke, Department of Defense, and numerous other agencies. He is statistical consultant for the journal *Headache: The Journal of Head and Face Pain* and statistical editor for the journal *Anesthesiology*. Key appointments have included serving as a member of the Behavioral Medicine: Interventions and Outcomes Study Section (National Institutes of Health), chair of the Methodology, Design, and Statistical Issues Section (American Headache Society), member of the Behavioral Clinical Trials Guidelines Workgroup (American Headache Society), and member of the Common Data Elements Working Group for Headache Clinical Trials (National Institute of Neurological Disorders and Stroke).

About the Cover Illustration

Title of Print: *Going Against the Migraine* by Enoch "Doyle" Jeter
The cover image is an etching done on a zinc plate, hand colored and printed by the artist. It was created as an original, limited edition print and commissioned as cover art for this volume.

Artist's Comment: *Although perhaps a bit over the top, I hope my depiction of what it feels like to suffer from a migraine captures those terrible moments so many of us sadly experience. Discussions with the authors (Don Penzien and others) were crucial in deciding on how to approach the image. My hat...and anvil...are off to them.*

About the artist: Enoch "Doyle" Jeter
- Born in Jena, Louisiana, USA
- Bachelor of Arts, Northeast Louisiana University, Monroe, Louisiana
- Master of Fine Arts, Highlands University, Las Vegas, New Mexico
- Printmaking Instructor and Artist in Residence, University of Louisiana–Monroe
- Public and private collections: USA, Ireland, Venezuela, Canada, Holland, Bali-Indonesia, Germany, Puerto Rico, etc.
- Numerous exhibitions, 1971 to present
- Artist's web site: http://www.enochdoylejeterart.com/

To enquire about ordering signed prints of the cover illustration (*Going Against the Migraine*), please contact the author at doyle@enochdoylejeterart.com. All other enquiries are also welcome.

Advances in Psychotherapy – Evidence-Based Practice

Series Editor

Danny Wedding, PhD, MPH, School of Medicine, American University of Antigua, St. Georges, Antigua

Associate Editors

Larry Beutler, PhD, Professor, Palo Alto University / Pacific Graduate School of Psychology, Palo Alto, CA

Kenneth E. Freedland, PhD, Professor of Psychiatry and Psychology, Washington University School of Medicine, St. Louis, MO

Linda C. Sobell, PhD, ABPP, Professor, Center for Psychological Studies, Nova Southeastern University, Ft. Lauderdale, FL

David A. Wolfe, PhD, RBC Chair in Children's Mental Health, Centre for Addiction and Mental Health, University of Toronto, ON

The basic objective of this series is to provide therapists with practical, evidence-based treatment guidance for the most common disorders seen in clinical practice – and to do so in a "reader-friendly" manner. Each book in the series is both a compact "how-to" reference on a particular disorder for use by professional clinicians in their daily work, as well as an ideal educational resource for students and for practice-oriented continuing education.

The most important feature of the books is that they are practical and easy to use: All are structured similarly and all provide a compact and easy-to-follow guide to all aspects that are relevant in real-life practice. Tables, boxed clinical "pearls," marginal notes, and summary boxes assist orientation, while checklists provide tools for use in daily practice.

Headache

Todd A. Smitherman
Department of Psychology, University of Mississippi, Oxford, MS

Donald B. Penzien
Department of Anesthesiology, Wake Forest School of Medicine,
Winston-Salem, NC

Jeanetta C. Rains
Center for Sleep Evaluation, Elliot Hospital, Manchester, NH

Robert A. Nicholson
Mercy Clinic Headache Center/Mercy Health Research, Mercy Health,
St. Louis, MO

Timothy T. Houle
Department of Anesthesiology, Wake Forest School of Medicine,
Winston-Salem, NC

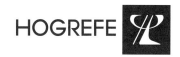

Library of Congress Cataloging in Publication
is available via the Library of Congress Marc Database under the
Library of Congress Control Number 2014947999

Library and Archives Canada Cataloguing in Publication
Smitherman, Todd A., 1977-, author
      Headache / Todd A. Smitherman, Department of Psychology, University of Mississippi, Oxford, MS, Donald B. Penzien, Department of Anesthesiology, Wake Forest School of Medicine, Winston-Salem, NC, Jeanetta C. Rains, Center for Sleep Evaluation, Elliot Hospital, Manchester, NH, Robert A. Nicholson, Mercy Clinic Headache Center/Mercy Health Research, Mercy Health, St. Louis, MO, Timothy T. Houle, Department of Anesthesiology, Wake Forest School of Medicine, Winston-Salem, NC.

(Advances in psychotherapy--evidence based practice series ; volume 30)
Includes bibliographical references.
Issued in print and electronic formats.
ISBN 978-0-88937-328-0 (pbk.).--ISBN 978-1-61676-328-2 (pdf).--
ISBN 978-1-61334-328-9 (html)

      1. Headache. 2. Headache--Treatment. I. Penzien, Donald B., 1957-, author II. Rains, Jeanetta C., 1963-, author III. Nicholson, Robert A., 1971-, author IV. Houle, Timothy T., 1974-, author V. Title. VI. Series: Advances in psychotherapy--evidence-based practice ; v. 30

RC392.S65 2014   616.8'491   C2014-905388-6
                                         C2014-905389-4

© 2015 by Hogrefe Publishing
http://www.hogrefe.com

PUBLISHING OFFICES
USA: Hogrefe Publishing Corporation, 38 Chauncy Street, Suite 1002, Boston, MA 02111
                     Phone (866) 823-4726, Fax (617) 354-6875; E-mail customerservice@hogrefe-publishing.com
EUROPE: Hogrefe Publishing GmbH, Merkelstr. 3, 37085 Göttingen, Germany
                     Phone +49 551 99950-0, Fax +49 551 99950-425; E-mail publishing@hogrefe.com

SALES & DISTRIBUTION
USA: Hogrefe Publishing, Customer Services Department,
                     30 Amberwood Parkway, Ashland, OH 44805
                     Phone (800) 228-3749, Fax (419) 281-6883; E-mail customerservice@hogrefe.com
UK: Hogrefe Publishing c/o Marston Book Services Ltd, 160 Eastern Ave.,
                     Milton Park, Abingdon, OX14 4SB, UK
                     Phone +44 1235 465577, Fax +44 1235 465556; E-mail direct.orders@marston.co.uk
EUROPE: Hogrefe Publishing, Merkelstr. 3, 37085 Göttingen, Germany
                     Phone +49 551 99950-0, Fax +49 551 99950-425; E-mail publishing@hogrefe.com

OTHER OFFICES
CANADA: Hogrefe Publishing, 660 Eglinton Ave. East, Suite 119-514, Toronto, Ontario, M4G 2K2
SWITZERLAND: Hogrefe Publishing, Länggass-Strasse 76, CH-3000 Bern 9

Hogrefe Publishing
Incorporated and registered in the Commonwealth of Massachusetts, USA, and in Göttingen, Lower Saxony, Germany

Printed and bound in the USA

ISBN 978-0-88937-328-0 (print), ISBN 978-1-61676-328-2 (pdf), ISBN 978-1-61334-328-9 (epub)
http://doi.org/10.1027/00328-000

Preface

This book describes the conceptualization, assessment, and empirically supported treatment of headache from a behavioral perspective. Though headache most certainly is at its core a neurobiological phenomenon, a large and ever-growing body of research indicates that behavioral factors (e.g., stress, psychiatric comorbidities, coping skills, cognitions) play an integral role in the onset and maintenance of headache disorders over time. Many mental health providers encounter headache as a common and disabling comorbidity among their psychiatric patients but lack the knowledge of how to effectively work with headache patients. Hundreds of studies over the past 4 decades have amply established the efficacy of behavioral therapies for headache disorders as well as the relevance of psychological/behavioral factors in headache. This book reviews the relevant psychological factors and describes how to implement efficacious behavioral interventions for headache within clinical practice settings. The intended audience is principally mental/behavioral health practitioners and trainees who want to know how to implement these interventions with their patients. This volume is also useful for other health care professionals wishing to supplement routine medical treatment of headache patients with empirically supported behavioral strategies. Basic familiarity with psychological principles of behavior change is assumed.

This book is divided into five chapters. Chapter 1 describes the most common primary headache disorders, differentiating migraine and tension-type headache from each other and from other headache disorders, reviewing common comorbid conditions, and outlining empirically supported assessment strategies. Chapter 2 gives an overview of the pathophysiology of migraine and the behavioral conceptualization of headache. Chapter 3 presents a framework for conducting a diagnostic assessment and identifying factors affecting a patient's suitability for and response to treatment. Chapter 4 presents a step-by-step, manual-type guide to implementing the various interventions. This chapter includes a review of treatment efficacy and mechanisms of action, variations on the standard format of delivery, and strategies for addressing common problems in treatment. Chapter 5 provides a broad summary of the prior chapters. The Appendix provides a set of useful assessment and treatment forms and handouts.

Although tension-type headache is the most common of the primary headache disorders, migraine is the most common diagnosis among those who present for headache treatment within clinical settings. As such, the bulk of this volume focuses on migraine and migraine-specific comorbidities. However, the relevance and adaptation of assessment and treatment strategies for tension-type headache are integrated into various sections when appropriate and supported empirically. Although behavioral interventions are highly efficacious for children with headache, the primary focus herein is on adults with headache disorders; considerations for child and adolescent patients are incorporated when appropriate. This volume outlines multiple behavioral strategies and interventions but is not intended as a one-size-fits-all, cookbook-type manual. The clinician is instead encouraged to individualize and select interventions tailored to patient needs, resources, and other considerations. As such, this volume is intended to provide a structured approach that can be adapted across multiple clinical contexts and among a variety of headache patients.

Acknowledgments

We would like to acknowledge series editor Dr. Danny Wedding, associate editor Dr. Kenneth Freedland, and Mr. Robert Dimbleby of Hogrefe Publishing. Their guidance and wisdom throughout the process of assembling this volume, the first major book on this topic in over 20 years, was invaluable. We are grateful to our undergraduate and graduate academic mentors: Drs. Stephen Chew, Dudley McGlynn, and Donald Penzien (T.A.S.); Drs. James Motiff, Kenneth Holroyd, and Thomas Creer (D.B.P.); Drs. James Snyder and Robert Zettle (J.C.R.); Drs. Sandra Gramling, Justin Nash, Kenneth Holroyd, and Frank Andrasik (R.A.N.); and Drs. Lori Rokicki and James Eisenach (T.T.H.). They taught us, challenged us, and instilled in us a commitment to scientifically informed practice and a love and respect for the field of behavioral medicine.

We wish to extend our utmost gratitude to coauthor Dr. Donald Penzien, who directly trained three of us (T.A.S., J.C.R., and T.T.H.), who mentored our early headache careers, and whose experimental and clinical contributions to behavioral medicine are unparalleled.

We are grateful also to our colleagues and students at the University of Mississippi, University of Mississippi Medical Center, Elliott Hospital, Mercy Clinic Headache Center/Mercy Health Research, and Wake Forest School of Medicine.

The concepts and strategies included herein reflect our combined experience of nearly 100 years in seeing headache patients and conducting headache research. We are grateful to every patient and research participant who has entrusted us with your pain, suffering, and experiences – for in your strength and sharing these pages were born. You inspired us to attend to aspects of your pain beyond the symptoms alone. This book is dedicated to you.

To our families – your love and support made our careers, and ultimately this volume, possible.

Dedications

To my parents, Johnny and Kathy, for an unwavering foundation of support and love. (T.A.S.)

To my daughter, Caitlin Penzien – the joy of my life. And to the many trainees and colleagues who have served as treasured friends and collaborators over the years, including Dr. Jeanetta Rains, Dr. Tim Houle, Dr. Todd Smitherman, and Dr. Ken Holroyd, to name only just a few. (D.B.P.)

To my parents, Paul and Ellen Rains, for a lifetime of love and encouragement. (J.C.R.)

To my parents, Don and Judy. To my amazing daughters, Ashtyn and Ansley – you both bring a smile to my heart every day. To my wife, Hilari – your unconditional love, support, and friendship makes me fall more in love with you every day. (R.A.N.)

To my mother, Mary Lou. To my brothers, Jeff and Chris – I have written a book and you have not. To Dr. Todd Smitherman – Thank you for your herculean efforts in the writing of this book. (T.T.H.)

Table of Contents

1

Description

1.1 Terminology

Criteria for the diagnosis of headache disorders are outlined in the third edition of the *International Classification of Headache Disorders* (ICHD-3; Headache Classification Committee of the International Headache Society, 2013). *Migraine without aura* (ICHD-3 1.1; *International Classification of Diseases,* 10th ed. [ICD-10] G43.0) was known previously as common migraine. *Migraine with aura* (ICHD-3 1.2, ICD-10 G43.1) was known previously as classic or classical migraine. *Tension-type headache* (TTH; ICHD-3 2.1–2.4, ICD-10 G44.2) has in the past been termed muscle contraction headache, stress headache, and ordinary headache. These "primary" headache disorders represent the most common headache conditions that are not directly attributable to secondary abnormalities.

The term *episodic* is applied to most migraine (episodic migraine [EM]) and TTH (episodic tension-type headache [ETTH]) diagnoses and formally refers to headache attacks that occur fewer than 15 days per month. In rare cases in which patients report experiencing attacks on 15 or more days per month, a diagnosis of either *chronic migraine* (CM; ICHD-3 1.3, ICD-10 G43.3) or *chronic TTH* (CTTH; ICHD-3 2.3, ICD-10 G44.2) is warranted, depending upon which headache type is predominant. The term *chronic* is somewhat of a misnomer – although a history of over 3 months is required for a diagnosis of CM or CTTH, chronic headache disorders are those in which attacks occur with high *frequency* (≥ 15 days/month).

> *Chronic* headache occurs on 15 or more days per month

1.2 Definition

Migraine is classified in the ICHD-3 as a neurological disorder characterized by recurrent headache attacks lasting hours or sometimes days (4–72 hr if untreated); its prototypical feature is severe head pain that is distributed unilaterally (on one side of the head), has a pulsating/throbbing quality, and interferes with usual activities. Migraine must also be accompanied by (1) nausea, (2) vomiting, or (3) sensitivity to *both* light (photophobia) and sound (phonophobia) (see Table 1). A significant minority of migraine patients experience *aura* symptoms, or temporary alterations in vision, sensation, or speech that typically precede but may occur simultaneously with the onset of

> **Migraine is severe, one-sided, throbbing head pain with nausea and/or sensitivity to light and sound**

> **Migraine aura is usually visual in nature**

Table 1
Diagnostic Criteria for Migraine

Migraine without aura

A. At least 5 attacks fulfilling all criteria B–D
B. Headache attacks lasting 4–72 hours (untreated or unsuccessfully treated)
C. Headache has at least two of the following characteristics:
   1. Unilateral location
   2. Pulsating quality
   3. Moderate or severe pain intensity
   4. Aggravation by or causing avoidance of routine physical activity (e.g., walking or climbing stairs)
D. During headache at least one of the following:
   1. Nausea and/or vomiting
   2. Photophobia and phonophobia
E. Not better accounted for by another ICHD-3 diagnosis

Migraine with aura

A. At least 2 attacks fulfilling all criteria B and C
B. One or more of the following fully reversible aura symptoms:
   1. visual
   2. sensory
   3. speech and/or language
   4. motor
   5. brainstem
   6. retinal
C. At least two of the following four characteristics:
   1. At least one aura symptom spreads gradually over ≥ 5 min, and/or two or more symptoms occur in succession
   2. Each individual aura symptom lasts 5–60 min
   3. At least one aura symptom is unilateral[a]
   4. The aura is accompanied, or followed within 60 min, by headache
D. Not better accounted for by another ICHD-3 diagnosis, and transient ischemic attack has been excluded

Note. [a]Aphasia is always regarded a unilateral symptom.
Excerpted from the ICHD-3 beta diagnostic criteria for migraine without aura (Code 1.1) and migraine with aura (Code 1.2): Headache Classification Committee of the International Headache Society. (2013). The International Classification of Headache Disorders (3rd ed., beta version). *Cephalalgia, 33*, 629–808. © SAGE. Reprinted with permission.

headache. Most commonly, migraine aura is experienced as a slowly evolving but temporary visual distortion (e.g., seeing lights, spots, zigzag lines) that lasts less than an hour and is followed quickly by onset of headache and other migraine symptoms. Migraine attacks in children are often of shorter duration than in adults (commonly < 4 hr), and the pain is often distributed bilaterally.

TTH is a recurrent headache disorder typically characterized by symptoms opposite those of migraine: mild to moderate pain that is distributed bilaterally across the head, which is nonpulsatile, does not interfere with activity, and is not accompanied by nausea, vomiting, or both photophobia and phonophobia (see Table 2). The duration of TTH may be as short as 30 min or as long as 1 week.

Tension-type headache symptoms are commonly the opposite those of migraine

Table 2
Diagnostic Criteria for Tension-Type Headache (TTH)

A. At least 10 episodes occurring on 1–14 days per month on average for
   > 3 months (≥ 12 and < 180 days per year) and fulfilling all criteria B–D
B. Lasting from 30 min to 7 days
C. At least two of the following four characteristics:
   1. Bilateral location
   2. Pressing or tightening (non-pulsating) quality
   3. Mild or moderate intensity
   4. Not aggravated by routine physical activity such as walking or climbing
      stairs
D. Both of the following:
   1. No nausea or vomiting
   2. No more than one of photophobia or phonophobia
E. Not better accounted for by another ICHD-3 diagnosis

Note. Excerpted from the ICHD-3 beta diagnostic criteria for frequent episodic TTH (Code 2.2): Headache Classification Committee of the International Headache Society. (2013). The International Classification of Headache Disorders (3rd ed., beta version). *Cephalalgia, 33,* 629–808. © SAGE. Reprinted with permission.

1.3 Epidemiology

Most people will experience headache at some point in life, and nearly half of the population (46%) has a headache disorder currently (Stovner et al., 2007). In fact, data from the 2010 Global Burden of Disease Study indicate that tension-type headache and migraine are, respectively, the second and third most common medical conditions worldwide (Vos et al., 2012). Studies adhering to ICHD diagnostic criteria document that migraine affects approximately 12% of Americans each year (Lipton et al., 2007) and 3 out of 10 in their lifetime (Stewart, Wood, Reed, Roy, & Lipton, 2008), although somewhat higher prevalence rates have been obtained from national surveillance studies (Smitherman, Burch, Sheikh, & Loder, 2013). Migraine differentially affects women (three times more often than men; 17.1% vs. 5.6% for 1-year prevalence, 43% vs. 18% for lifetime incidence) and is more prevalent among Whites than individuals of other races, as well as those of lower (vs. higher) socioeconomic status (SES; Lipton et al., 2007; Stewart et al., 2008). Prevalence is highest during young-to-middle adulthood, peaking between ages 30 and 39 (28.1% of women, 9.0% of men) and declining thereafter, being least common among those ages 60 and above. Migraine thus occurs most commonly during the peak years of adult productivity. Two thirds of migraine cases occur without regular aura symptoms. Despite the impact of migraine, approximately one third of migraineurs have never consulted a physician about their condition and of those who have, 40% remain with their condition undiagnosed (Lipton, Stewart, & Simon, 1998). Considered together, these statistics indicate that over half of individuals with migraine never receive a diagnosis.

Migraine is frequently underdiagnosed and thus undertreated

ETTH is the most common headache type among the general population, affecting roughly 40% of Americans each year (Schwartz, Stewart,

Simon, & Lipton, 1998; Stovner et al., 2007). ETTH will affect half or more of Americans in their lifetime. As with migraine, prevalence of ETTH is greater among women than men, higher among White Americans than Black Americans, and peaks between ages 30 and 39. Unlike migraine, however, the sex discrepancy in ETTH prevalence is much less striking (5:4 female to male ratio), and ETTH occurs most frequently among those of higher education and income levels. CM and CTTH each affect approximately 2% of the population each year (Lipton, Bigal, Hamelsky, & Scher, 2008) and, like their episodic counterparts, are more common among women than men.

1.4   Course and Prognosis

Migraine is conceptualized as a chronic *disease*, not merely a severe headache

Migraine is now recognized as a disorder involving far more than head pain itself and includes sensitivity to headache between attacks, cortical abnormalities, associated neurological symptoms, and impairments in functioning and quality of life both during and between attacks. As with other chronic conditions (e.g., obesity, cardiovascular disease, cancer), migraine is indisputably associated with both biological and environmental risk factors, and thus management of associated lifestyle factors is fundamental to optimal care.

The majority of migraineurs have 1–4 days with migraine per month and experience substantial functional impairment during attacks, including the need for bed rest or restricted activity, and interference with home and occupational obligations. Indeed, migraine ranks as the eighth leading cause of disability worldwide and alone accounts for over half of the years lived with disability from all neurological disorders (Vos et al., 2012). Most ETTH sufferers experience 1–3 headaches per month. Although TTH can be disabling, TTH is usually accompanied by less functional impairment than is typical of migraine. The high prevalence of ETTH nevertheless confers significant cumulative direct and indirect burdens to society.

Most migraine and TTH conditions affecting adults emerge in late adolescence or early adulthood as episodic conditions; 75% of migraineurs experience onset prior to age 35 (Stewart et al., 2008). The majority of EM and ETTH sufferers can manage their headaches with lifestyle accommodations and occasional use of over-the-counter remedies, without intervention by a physician. Many of these individuals will experience a reduction or cessation of headache within several months or years.

Headache "chronification" occurs in a minority of individuals

Among a minority of individuals, EM and ETTH progress in frequency over time to become chronic in nature (i.e., headache on ≥ 15 days per month). For more than a decade, the nature and predictors of headache progression and remission have been under increasingly intense scrutiny by headache researchers (Penzien, Rains, & Lipton, 2008). This research has revealed that observed increases in headache frequency are sometimes attributable to risk factors such as overusing analgesic medications, psychiatric comorbidities, and development or exacerbation of concurrent medical conditions such as obesity (Scher, Midgette, & Lipton, 2008). This pattern of "headache chronification" (progressing from an episodic to chronic frequency) is estimated to occur among approximately 3% of headache sufferers each year (Scher,

Stewart, Ricci, & Lipton, 2003), although actual rates of chronification may be somewhat lower (Houle, Turner, Smitherman, Penzien, & Lipton, 2013). High-frequency headaches also revert from CM to EM or from CTTH to ETTH at a much higher rate than chronification occurs. Not surprisingly, a higher frequency of headache is associated with higher headache-related disability, more frequent medical visits, and a poorer long-term prognosis. Most patients with CM or CTTH suffer for years with headache and, although the frequency of their attacks may fluctuate over time, they rarely become completely headache-free.

1.5   Differential Diagnosis

Primary headache disorders are diagnosed by their phenotypic presentations, and therefore differentiating between migraine and TTH is usually straightforward. As a general rule, most treatment-seeking patients with recurrent severe headaches accompanied by nausea and substantial functional impairment have migraine. Severe unilateral and pulsating pain that lasts for hours or days, interferes with activity, and is accompanied by nausea and sensitivity to light and sound are prototypical symptoms of migraine, although many patients will not present with all of these symptoms. A helpful mnemonic for distinguishing migraine from other headaches is the P.O.U.N.D.ing algorithm (see box below). The presence of three or more of these five features makes a migraine diagnosis highly probable (Detsky et al., 2006).

Recurrent severe headaches that impair functioning are usually migraines

P.O.U.N.D. is a useful mnemonic for migraine symptoms

P.O.U.N.D.ing Algorithm for Identifying Migraine (Detsky et al., 2006)

Pulsating
4–72 h**O**ur duration (if left untreated)
Unilateral
Nausea
Disabling

By contrast, TTH attacks are typically the opposite of migraine: They involve less severe pain that is typically distributed bilaterally, they are described as a constant tight pressure (nonpulsatile), and they lack the impairment and accompanying symptoms of migraine. Occasionally, a patient will present with some headache attacks consistent with migraine and others with TTH, in which case both diagnoses are assigned. Other headache conditions that may be mistaken for migraine are discussed below and should be ruled out before beginning treatment.

1.5.1   Cluster Headache

Cluster headache is a rare headache disorder (0.1% lifetime prevalence) that affects men more often than women and is characterized by excruciating pain commonly centered around the orbital socket. Cluster headache is typi-

Cluster headache is a very rare headache condition that affects men more often than women

cally accompanied by facial swelling, perspiration, and tearing of the eye on the same side of the head as the pain. The term *cluster* refers to the fact that headache episodes tend to cluster together in time and may occur up to several times a day. Cluster periods can last for weeks, months, or longer, and are then followed by a period of remission until another recurrence. Characteristics that differentiate cluster headache from migraine are the former's high predominance among males (4:1 to 5:1 male to female ratio), briefer attack duration (< 3 hr), common localization to the orbital socket, visibly obvious swelling or tearing around the eye, greater pain severity, and clustered patterning of attacks. Unlike migraineurs who tend to withdraw to a darkened, quiet place and lie down, many cluster patients shun resting and instead pace the floor because the pain is so extreme.

1.5.2   Medication Overuse Headache

Overuse of analgesic medications is the most common precipitant of chronic migraine

Overuse of acute headache medications is the most common variable known to precipitate the development of a chronic headache condition. Medication overuse headache (MOH) is diagnosed when an individual experiences chronic headache (≥ 15 days/month) and has used acute migraine medications (analgesics, ergotamine, triptans) for at least 10 days per month (for opioids, ergotamine, triptans, combination analgesics, or multiple drug classes) or at least 15 days per month (in the case of simple analgesics) for more than 3 months. The headaches typically worsen during the period of medication overuse. In cases in which the patient meets criteria for both CM and MOH, both diagnoses should be applied (see Table 3).

In clinical practice, medication overuse should be suspected and assessed in any patient reporting chronic headaches (15 or more days/month), even among those who do not identify their own medication use as excessive. Opioid analgesics are the most common culprits, but MOH can occur even among frequent users of over-the-counter pain medications (e.g., aspirin, acetaminophen). Daily use of medications approved by the US Food and Drug Administration (FDA) for migraine prevention is not a recognized cause of

Table 3
Diagnostic Criteria for Medication Overuse Headache (MOH)

A. Headache occurring on ≥ 15 days per month in a patient with a preexisting headache disorder
B. Regular overuse[a] for > 3 months of one or more drugs that can be taken for acute and/or symptomatic treatment of headache
C. Not better accounted for by another ICHD-3 diagnosis

Note. [a]Overuse defined as use of opioids, ergotamine, triptans, combination analgesics, or multiple drug classes at least 10 days per month, or use of simple analgesics at least 15 days per month.
Excerpted from the ICHD-3 beta diagnostic criteria for MOH (Code 8.2): Headache Classification Committee of the International Headache Society. (2013). The International Classification of Headache Disorders (3rd ed., beta version). *Cephalalgia, 33*, 629–808. © SAGE. Reprinted with permission.

MOH. The headaches in MOH often have migrainous features but also may share some features of TTH.

Many patients are unaware that frequent use of acute medications can inadvertently worsen headache over time. When MOH is suspected, treatment typically requires supervised medical withdrawal from the overused medication(s), sometimes in an inpatient setting. This process usually results in initial exacerbation of headache over the first several days, with gradual improvement thereafter.

1.5.3   Posttraumatic Headache

Posttraumatic headache (PTHA) is diagnosed when an unremitting or recurrent headache disorder develops (i.e., begins anew or constitutes a substantive change in a preexisting headache pattern) in temporal proximity following a head, neck, or brain injury. Observable physical or neurological signs or symptoms may or may not be present; in fact, they are often absent. The PTHA label is applied regardless of the characteristics of the headache itself, which often vary across individuals. Any headache that develops within a week of a head injury (or after regaining consciousness from a head injury) should be considered PTHA until determined otherwise. Fortunately, PTHA generally improves within a few months of onset. By convention, once PTHA has been present for 6 months, it is termed chronic: The longer the chronicity of PTHA, the more refractory it becomes. Although conventional wisdom holds that patients with chronic PTHA may not prove as responsive to behavioral interventions as those with migraine or TTH, empirical evidence and clinical experience supporting that impression are limited.

1.5.4   "Sinus Headache"

Both patients and physicians alike often mistakenly attribute head pain in the facial region (particularly the nose and eyes) or that accompanied by nasal congestion to inflammation of the paranasal sinuses. Many, if not most, of these patients in fact meet criteria for migraine that is triggered by weather/seasonal changes or accompanied by autonomic nasal symptoms (Schreiber et al., 2004). The presence of clear symptoms of acute rhinosinusitis is the most important determinant for differential diagnosis.

Many patients who attribute their headaches to sinus problems in fact have migraine

1.5.5   Menstrual Migraine

Many premenopausal women experience migraine attacks 1–2 days before or after the onset of menstrual bleeding. Some women have migraine attacks only around menstruation (*pure menstrual migraine*; ICHD-3 A1.1.1), while others have migraine attacks also during other times in the month (*menstrually related migraine*; ICHD-II A1.1.2). Migraine attacks associated with menstruation usually do not include aura symptoms.

Migraine attacks often coincide with menses

1.6   Diagnostic Red Flags

Patients with prototypical migraine symptoms and a normal neurological exam very rarely have significant abnormalities upon neuroimaging

The overwhelming majority of headaches are benign and *not* attributable to progressive or life-threatening intracranial pathology (e.g., neoplasm, hydrocephalus, subarachnoid hemorrhage). For patients who have recurrent but typical migrainous or TTH presentations and a normal neurological examination, neuroimaging including magnetic resonance imaging (MRI) and computed tomography (CT) is usually unwarranted, as fewer than 1% of such patients will evidence meaningful intracranial pathology upon imaging (Sempere et al., 2005). The strongest predictor of significant intracranial pathology is any abnormal finding during a routine neurological examination. The presence of neurological abnormalities and other "red flags" should raise suspicion of intracranial pathology, and referral to a physician for medical evaluation and possible neuroimaging is recommended. A popular mnemonic for red flags warranting medical evaluation is "SNOOP" (Dodick, 2003; see Table 4).

Table 4
SNOOP Algorithm for Headache Red Flags

Systemic symptoms or disease
    Fever, chills, weight changes
    Chronic medical comorbidity (malignancy, immunocompromised)

Neurological signs or symptoms
    Abnormal neurological exam, altered mental state, confusion, seizures

Onset is sudden and severe
    "Worst headache of my life" that peaks within minutes[a]

Onset in a patient over 40

Pattern change in headache presentation
    Current headache is of different type or much more frequent than prior history
    Headache is never-ending versus prior history

Note. [a]Requires urgent medical investigation (regardless of other features). Based on Dodick, 2003.

1.7   Comorbidities

Migraine is associated with increased rates of other comorbid disorders

The burden and impact of primary headache disorders are compounded by the presence of other disorders that commonly co-occur with them. Comorbid psychiatric disorders, pain conditions, and other chronic medical conditions are observed more commonly among both migraine and nonmigrainous headache sufferers than among individuals without headache (Saunders, Merikangas, Low, Von Korff, & Kessler, 2008). The likelihood and severity of comorbidities increase proportionally with headache frequency. These comorbid disorders increase disability (Saunders et al., 2008) and complicate the treatment and prognosis of headache patients. Many also represent modifiable risk factors for the development of headache chronification (Dodick, 2009; Smitherman, Rains, & Penzien, 2009) and MOH (Radat et al., 2005).

1.7.1 Depression

Depression has long been recognized as a common comorbidity among head-ache patients, and epidemiological studies confirm that migraineurs are two to four times more likely to suffer from major depressive disorder (MDD) than are individuals without migraine (Breslau, 1998; Hamelsky & Lipton, 2006). Lifetime prevalence of MDD among migraineurs ranges from 21% to 32%, although prevalence as high as 57% has been observed among individuals with CM (Breslau, 1998; Juang, Wang, Fuh, Lu, & Su, 2000). The relationship between migraine and depression is bidirectional in nature (Breslau, Lipton, Stewart, Schultz, & Welch, 2003), such that having either condition increases one's risk of developing the other. Depression is thus not simply a reaction to living with a recurrent headache condition. Patients with CTTH also have increased rates of MDD (Heckman & Holroyd, 2006).

1.7.2 Anxiety Disorders

Although migraine studies on depression outnumber those on anxiety dis-orders by a ratio of 2:1 (Smitherman, Penzien, & Maizels, 2008), anxiety disorders are nearly twice as common among migraine sufferers as depres-sion. Approximately 50% of all migraine sufferers will meet criteria for an anxiety disorder at some point (Breslau, 1998), the most common of which are panic disorder, generalized anxiety disorder (GAD), and phobias (Radat & Swendsen, 2005; Smitherman, Kolivas, & Bailey, 2013). Anxiety disor-ders may precede or follow onset of migraine. Among patients with both depressive *and* anxiety disorders, onset of anxiety usually precedes onset of migraine, which in turn precedes depression. As with depression, rates of anxiety disorders are highest among those with chronic (vs. episodic) migraine and TTH.

Anxiety disorders are more common than depression among migraine patients

Bidirectional relationships between mood/anxiety disorders and migraine imply shared mechanisms, although research on mechanistic underpinnings is in its infancy. The most likely contributors are serotonergic dysfunction, sensi-tization of the central nervous system (CNS), and hormonal influences, though these factors interact and none is likely to be the sole contributor (Baskin & Smitherman, 2009).

Both migraine and affective conditions are associated with reduced seroto-nergic availability and respond to pharmacological agents that increase central serotonin levels (Hamel, 2007). Specifically, selective serotonin (5HT) ago-nists (i.e., triptans) are the mainstay of current acute treatments for migraine, and selective serotonin reuptake inhibitors (SSRIs) are the agents-of-choice for mood and anxiety disorders. Prolonged sensitization of the CNS, par-ticularly sensory/emotional neural networks, is likely involved among patients with chronic headache subforms (Baskin & Smitherman, 2009). Ovarian hormone changes are implicated because affective disorders and migraine are much more common among women than men and because dramatic declines in estrogen (e.g., during the late luteal phase of the menstrual cycle, the post-partum period, and during perimenopause) often trigger episodes of these conditions (Martin & Behbehani, 2006).

1.7.3   Other Psychiatric Comorbidities

Although other psychiatric disorders have been studied less frequently than depression and anxiety, migraineurs also appear to be at significantly increased risk for bipolar spectrum disorders (Breslau, 1998; Saunders et al., 2008). Recent data indicate an association between migraine in adulthood and a history of childhood abuse/neglect (Tietjen & Peterlin, 2011), although this relationship may be mediated by development of posttraumatic stress disorder (Smitherman & Kolivas, 2013). At present it is unclear whether migraineurs are at increased risk for substance use disorders, as existing studies have produced largely mixed findings. Individuals in inpatient treatment for chronic headache, in particular, have significantly increased rates of personality disorders, most commonly those with dramatic and anxious features (Lake, Saper, & Hamel, 2009). Migraineurs also are at increased risk for suicide attempts, even after controlling for psychiatric comorbidities (Breslau, Schultz, Lipton, Peterson, & Welch, 2012).

1.7.4   Insomnia and Other Disturbances of Sleep

Headache may result from, be aggravated by, or contribute to sleep disturbance, and both too little and too much sleep can trigger migraine (Rains & Poceta, 2006). In addition, many migraineurs have disrupted sleep schedules because migraine attacks often prompt bed rest. Obstructive sleep apnea and other sleep-related breathing disorders associated with hypoxemia or hypercapnia may contribute to headache among individuals with morning headaches or chronic headaches. Patients at risk for sleep-disordered breathing should be advised to consult with their physician to determine whether referral to a sleep medicine specialist is needed.

Although a variety of sleep disorders are more common among those with headache than those without, insomnia is the most prevalent sleep disorder among treatment-seeking patients with migraine or TTH (Kelman & Rains, 2005). Generally, insomnia refers to recurrent difficulty initiating or maintaining sleep, short duration of sleep, or nonrestorative sleep, which results in daytime functional impairment (e.g., fatigue, difficulty concentrating, irritability). Research diagnostic criteria for insomnia have been operationalized as sleep onset latency > 30 min, awakenings > 30 min after falling asleep, total sleep time < 6 hr, or subjective complaints of nonrestorative sleep in the context of daytime impairment.

Insomnia is an extremely common comorbidity, particularly among chronic headache sufferers

At least half of all headache clinic patients will meet the diagnostic criteria for insomnia. As with other comorbidities, the prevalence of insomnia increases with headache frequency, such that the overwhelming majority of chronic migraineurs experience insomnia, often on a daily basis. Treating the comorbid sleep disorder directly often reduces the frequency of headache (Calhoun & Ford, 2007).

1.7.5   Obesity

Perhaps because it is a proinflammatory state, obesity is associated with increased frequency of headache. Headache frequency increases proportionally with body mass index (BMI), such that individuals who are obese (BMI of 30–34) or morbidly obese (BMI ≥ 35) are, respectively, 2.9 and 5.7 times more likely than those of normal weight to have headache on 10 or more days per month (Bigal, Liberman, & Lipton, 2006). Similarly, obesity is a risk factor for progression from episodic to chronic headache frequency (Scher et al., 2003).

1.7.6   Cardiovascular Disease

Although an individual migraine attack itself rarely triggers a stroke, migraine may be associated with increased risk for stroke (Bigal et al., 2010; Schürks et al., 2009). Risk is highest among women and those with aura symptoms, and increases further with cigarette smoking and use of oral contraceptives (particularly contraceptives containing high doses of estrogen).

1.8   Headache Triggers

Headache "triggers" are personal or environmental stimuli that precipitate an individual headache attack. Importantly, failure to address triggering or exacerbating factors is one of the most common reasons for failure of headache treatment (Lipton, Silberstein, Saper, Bigal, & Goadsby, 2003). Nearly all of the major headache triggers have strong behavioral components, and thus identification of relevant triggers provides multiple opportunities for behavioral intervention. Problematically, most research on headache triggers has relied on retrospective self-report rather than direct experimental manipulation of potential triggers. Table 5 lists the percentage of headache clinic patients endorsing various triggers across three major survey studies. The top triggers across self-reported studies are stress, menstruation, dietary factors (e.g., skipping meals, fasting), and sleep disturbance (e.g., insufficient sleep, irregular sleep/wake schedule, too much sleep), three of which have substantive behavioral influences. Other commonly reported triggers include weather changes, exercise, odors, and noises, although experimental studies have not always verified the potency of these triggers (see Table 5).

Although triggers are usually considered independently of one another, they are unlikely to act in isolation, and different individuals will usually have differing thresholds for headache onset. An ambitious prospective study of triggers analyzed 28,325 days of daily headache diary data collected from 327 migraineurs in Europe over a 3-month period (Wöber et al., 2007). These authors examined 116 variables pertaining to hormonal factors, psychological states, sleep, diet, activities, physical factors (e.g., hunger), environmental

Stress, menstruation, dietary factors, and sleep disturbance are the most common triggers of migraine

Table 5
Headache Triggers Across Three Major Survey Studies

Trigger	Kelman (2007)	Scharff et al. (1995)	Robbins (1994)
Stress	**80%**	72%	62%
Menstruation	65%	68%	50%
Fasting/missing meals	**57%**	**45%**	**40%**
Sleep disturbance	**50%**	.52%	**31%**
Weather	53%	46%	43%
Perfume or odor	44%	----	----
Neck pain	38%	----	----
Lights	38%	----	----
Alcohol	38%	35%	----
Smoking	36%	----	26%
Foods	27%	----	30%
Exercise	22%	----	----
Sexual activity	5%	----	----
Caffeine	----	14%	----

Note. Most common, modifiable self-reported headache triggers are shown in bold.

variables, and meteorological events. Among these numerous potential triggers, menstruation was identified as the most potent risk factor in predicting subsequent headache; occurrence of migraine or other headache was increased during all days of menstruation as well as during the 2 days preceding menstruation. Stress, neck tension, fatigue, noise, and odors also increased risk for migraine or other headaches. This study confirmed that myriad potential triggers act on the migraineur at any given time, including factors usually outside of awareness (e.g., atmospheric pressure changes, hormonal fluctuations). A recent study by our group also showed that high stress and poor sleep resulted in greater risk of subsequent headache than either trigger factor alone (Houle et al., 2012), again underscoring the interactive effect among various triggers.

Healthy lifestyle recommendations are useful for all headache patients

Healthy lifestyle recommendations to minimize stress, practice good sleep habits, and avoid skipping meals are encouraged for *all* patients, and many will benefit from more formal trigger management training as described later in this work (see Section 4.1.5).

1.9   Diagnostic Procedures and Documentation

Pain is a subjective experience that is not accessible to others. As such, and because consistent biomarkers for migraine and TTH have not yet been identified, assessment of headache in clinical practice relies on self-report methods.

1.9.1   Headache Self-Monitoring

Daily self-monitoring of headache is used as the principal means for assessing baseline headache activity and assessing progress in treatment. Self-monitoring using "headache diaries" should, at a minimum, quantify headache occurrence (frequency), peak severity, and duration (in hours) on a daily basis. More comprehensive forms also include options for monitoring related factors such as specific headache symptoms, current stress, sleep duration and/or quality, potential triggers, medication use, and, when appropriate, times of menstruation.

Recent advances in information technology have yielded electronic headache diaries (using local storage or via the Web) available as applications on smartphones and other handheld devices. These electronic diaries offer the benefits of real-time data collection, prompts for patient responses, and easy transmission to the provider. The information obtained can be used to identify specific targets for treatment as they occur and to provide feedback to the patient about potential headache precipitants (e.g., the most recent diary entry reveals that the patient did not practice good sleep hygiene the night before she had a headache). Furthermore, the electronic diary information can be used to conduct case-based time-series analyses for rapid assessment of treatment response (Borckardt et al., 2008).

Headache Frequency
Because migraine attacks often span multiple days, headache frequency should be quantified in *days* per week (or month) with headache, not the number of individual headache attacks. By convention, migraine or TTH occurring on 15 or more days per month is to be considered "chronic." Female patients should be queried as to whether their headaches coincide with menstruation.

Headache frequency is measured in days per week (or month) with headache, not the number of individual headache attacks

Headache Severity
The most common methods for assessing headache severity involve 4-point Likert-type, 6-point Likert-type, 11-point Likert-type, or visual analog scales. Each approach has advantages and disadvantages. We prefer a 0 to 10 Likert-type scale, in which 0 indicates "no pain" and 10 is indicative of "the worst pain imaginable," because it provides greater precision and opportunity for data analysis than rating scales with fewer options. Whichever severity scale is used, anchors must be provided for the corresponding numbers at the ends and middle of the scale, at a minimum. The patient should be reminded to report "peak" severity of the attack but to not be overly concerned with the exact rating she provides; a first impression is probably the best estimate. Table 6 describes the various options for quantifying headache severity.

We recommend quantifying pain severity on a 0–10 scale

Headache Duration
Headache duration is quantified as the number of hours the attack lasts. If the patient falls asleep with headache and wakes up without headache, duration should be assumed to be until waking.

Instructions for Self-Monitoring
We recommend having patients self-monitor their headache activity for (1) a period of 2–5 weeks prior to beginning treatment (but after the intake) and

Table 6
Assessing Headache Severity

Format	Response anchors for peak severity	Comments
4-point	0 = No headache 1 = Mild pain 2 = Moderate pain 3 = Severe pain	Often used in drug trials Limited for assessing change Psychometrically weaker than other options
6-point	0 = No pain 1 = Slight pain (only noticed when focused on it; no impact on daily activities) 2 = Mild pain (noticeable but did not interrupt concentration; little impact on activities) 3 = Moderate pain (noticeable but did not interrupt concentration; some impact on daily activities) 4 = Very painful (difficulty concentrating; significant impact on daily activities but able to perform simple tasks) 5 = Extreme pain (couldn't focus on anything else; unable to do any activities)	More precise than 4-point option Descriptors help frame the pain for the patient Descriptors may be distracting or unevenly weighted
11-point	0 = No headache 1, 2, 3, 4 5 = Moderate pain 6, 7, 8, 9 10 = Worst pain imaginable	Easily visualized by patients Useful for identifying small incremental improvements Between-patient variability in interpreting nonanchored numbers
Visual analog	Solid line between two anchor points (no pain vs. worst pain imaginable) Patients mark the point on the line corresponding to their pain	No restrictions on having to choose a specific number Confusing for some patients More time-consuming for the provider to score

(2) again after the last treatment session. Patients should return the provided self-monitoring forms at subsequent clinic visits for review. Self-monitoring continually throughout treatment may be indicated for some patients, but in general, frequent monitoring throughout treatment is often perceived as burdensome and even discouraging for some patients, as the effects of behavioral headache interventions often take weeks to become evident.

Because self-monitoring is perceived as an inconvenience for some patients, it is essential to provide a strong rationale for the importance of self-monitoring. This rationale should focus on the benefits of regular self-monitoring in tracking headache activity accurately, monitoring progress in treatment, and identifying potential triggers; the patient should be informed that self-monitoring should take no more than a few minutes each day. *The patient should be instructed to record headache activity at least two, and ideally four, times each day.* Recording should be spaced throughout the day and occur even if the patient is not having a headache at the time of recording. Adherence is facilitated by instructing the patient to pair self-monitoring with a routine daily activity such as mealtime or bedtime, or when taking medications. Others benefit from setting a reminder alarm to go off every 4 hr when awake, and many electronic headache diaries automatically prompt the user to record data at either preset or random intervals.

For patients who have difficulty with the longer Detailed Headache Self-Monitoring Form (see Appendix 1), or for those who are asked to complete self-monitoring daily throughout treatment, the once-daily Brief Headache Self-Monitoring Form is a viable alternative (see Appendix 2). Patient instructions for detailed self-monitoring are also provided (see Appendix 3).

Self-monitoring is integrated throughout the major components of behavioral headache therapies and incorporated into descriptions of the various behavioral treatment methods found later in this work (see Section 4.1).

> A minimum of 2 weeks, and preferably 4–5 weeks, of self-monitoring is used to quantify headache activity at baseline and after the last treatment session

> Pairing self-monitoring with a routine daily activity improves adherence

1.9.2   Headache Diagnostic Interviews

Structured diagnostic interviews are most useful for determining a patient's headache diagnosis according to ICHD diagnostic criteria. The Structured Diagnostic Interview for Headache-3 (SDIH-3) is recommended for this purpose and incorporates revisions to the original SDIH (Andrew, Penzien, Rains, Knowlton, & McAnulty, 1992) that ensure adherence to ICHD-3 diagnostic criteria. The SDIH-3 assesses the core diagnostic features of both migraine and TTH (episodic and chronic), and it includes additional appendix items to assess potential cluster headache, MOH, and PTHA. This structured interview is easy to use for individuals with a basic knowledge of headache and can be administered to most patients in approximately 20 min. The SDIH-3 and accompanying coding checklist are reprinted in the appendices (see Appendices 4 and 5).

> Structured headache interviews are the gold standard for establishing primary headache disorder diagnoses

1.9.3   Headache Questionnaires

Numerous self-report measures are available to assess the impact of headache on functioning. The two most commonly used and well-validated mea-

Table 7
Scoring and Interpretation of Measures Assessing Headache-Related Disability

	MIDAS		HIT-6
0–5	Little or no disability	< 50	Little or no disability
6–10	Mild disability	50–55	Mild disability
11–20	Moderate disability[a]	56–60	Moderate disability[a]
> 20	Severe disability[a]	> 60	Severe disability[a]

Note. HIT-6 = Headache Impact Test; MIDAS = Migraine Disability Assessment Questionnaire.
[a]Headaches are having a major impact on the patient's functioning.

sures of headache-related disability are the Migraine Disability Assessment Questionnaire (MIDAS; Stewart, Lipton, Kolodner, Liberman, & Sawyer, 1999) and the Headache Impact Test (HIT-6; Kosinski et al., 2003). The MIDAS includes five questions that quantify the number of days during the previous 3 months in which headaches have impaired the patient's ability to function at work/school, to perform household work, and to participate in leisure activities. Overall disability scores range from 0 to 270. Two additional questions provide data on headache frequency and severity but are not included in the overall disability score. The HIT-6 is a six-item Likert-type instrument that incorporates ratings of functional impairment, pain severity, and the emotional/cognitive impact of headache over the last 4 weeks. Scores range from 36 to 78. Interpretative guides for the MIDAS and HIT-6 are provided in Table 7. Other, more time-intensive options for assessing disability include the 25-item Headache Disability Inventory (HDI; Jacobson, Ramadan, Aggarwal, & Newman, 1994) and the 16-item Migraine-Specific Quality of Life Questionnaire (MSQL; Jhingran, Osterhouse, Miller, Lee, & Kirchdoerfer, 1998).

> **Locus of control and self-efficacy are psychological constructs of central importance**

Other self-report measures quantify psychological constructs of relevance (Nicholson, Houle, Rhudy, & Norton, 2007). Locus of control (LOC) for management of headache can be assessed with the Headache-Specific Locus of Control Scale (HSLC; Martin, Holroyd, & Penzien, 1990). The HSLC is a 33-item Likert-type scale that assesses beliefs regarding whether headache activity is influenced primarily by oneself, by medical professionals, or by fate. Self-efficacy (SE) in one's own ability to manage headache is assessed with the 25-item Headache Management Self-Efficacy Scale (HMSE-25; French et al., 2000). Both LOC and SE are discussed in detail later (see Section 2.4.2). For an overview of assessment of other psychological constructs of relevance to the headache patient, the interested reader is referred to Turner and Houle (2013).

1.9.4   Assessing Psychiatric Comorbidity

Verbal screening for comorbid depression or anxiety should focus on assessing the core diagnostic criteria of the *Diagnostic and Statistical Manual of Mental*

Disorders, 5th Edition (DSM-5; American Psychiatric Association, 2013) that are pathognomonic for the suspected condition. For depression, for instance, the core symptoms of interest are persistent depressed mood and anhedonia; for panic disorder, the focus is on recurrent panic attacks accompanied by fear of future attacks. Many migraine patients report "transdiagnostic symptoms," or physical symptoms characteristic of both migraine and affective disorders (e.g., sleep complaints, fatigue, trouble concentrating, irritability, nausea, and muscle tension; Holm, Penzien, Holroyd, & Brown, 1994). Disability manifesting as social withdrawal, avoidance, and inability to attend work or school may be attributable to impairment from headache, depression, anxiety, or even secondary gain in some circumstances. Focusing primarily on emotional and cognitive symptoms of suspected psychiatric disorders is therefore most useful in differentiating psychopathology from headache sequelae. Assessing the temporal onset of transdiagnostic symptoms in relation to headache onset and whether the symptoms occur exclusively during the headache episode are other helpful strategies.

> **Focusing on emotional and cognitive symptoms is useful in distinguishing psychiatric from headache-related symptoms**

The most appropriate self-report measures for psychiatric screening of headache sufferers are those that have been validated for use with medical patients. Although a number of different measures are likely appropriate to use in screening for psychopathology, the most common and well-validated measure of depression among headache patients is the nine-item depression module of the Patient Health Questionnaire (PHQ-9; Kroenke, Spitzer, & Williams, 2001). For anxiety symptomatology, the Generalized Anxiety Disorder seven-item scale (GAD-7; Spitzer, Kroenke, Williams, & Löwe, 2006) is used frequently. Although originally developed to assess GAD specifically, the GAD-7 also has demonstrated sensitivity and specificity in identifying other anxiety disorders such as posttraumatic stress disorder, panic disorder, and social phobia (Kroenke, Spitzer, Williams, Monahan, & Löwe, 2007). Scores of 10 or above on the PHQ-9 and GAD-7 are indicative of moderate or greater symptomatology and merit further evaluation. The PHQ-9 and GAD-7 are available at no cost online (see http://www.phqscreeners.com). Maizels, Smitherman, and Penzien (2006) review additional assessment measures and strategies for identifying these and other psychiatric comorbidities.

> **The PHQ-9 and GAD-7 are validated screeners for depression and anxiety, respectively**

1.9.5   Assessing Improvement Over Time

Improvement over time is typically gauged using headache frequency as the principal outcome of interest, as behavioral therapies are most useful in preventing (rather than aborting) headache episodes. Although many clinicians rely on global, retrospective self-reports of headache activity (e.g., verbal querying of previous headache activity at each session), this practice yields data that are often unreliable and influenced by self-report bias (Penzien et al., 1994). We strongly advocate for use of daily headache self-monitoring to obtain the most reliable and valid data pertaining to headache frequency, severity, and duration. For some patients, obtaining information from a collateral source (e.g., spouse, teacher, parent) is useful. Clinically meaningful improvements in headache frequency over the course of treatment, by convention, are those that represent 50% reductions from pretreatment values.

> **Headache frequency is the primary outcome variable**

Disability resulting from headache is an important outcome, especially among patients with chronic headache

Because the impact of headache extends well beyond pain itself, headache-related disability is also an outcome of utmost importance. Changes in headache-related disability should be tracked using the MIDAS or HIT-6, although the HIT-6 is perhaps most appropriate for assessing headache improvement frequently throughout treatment, as it includes a shorter recall interval (4-week vs. 90-day, respectively). Reductions in headache severity, headache duration, and frequency of acute medication use are secondary outcomes worthy of consideration, as are reductions in comorbid psychiatric conditions and utilization of medication or medical services, particularly for those with chronic headache subforms. Changes in depression and anxiety may be assessed easily on a weekly or biweekly (every two weeks) basis using the PHQ-9 or GAD-7, respectively. For many patients, improvements in disability, psychiatric symptomatology, and perceived control over headache may be every bit as meaningful as reductions in headache per se. In our experience, this is particularly true of patients with CM and CTTH.

2

Theories and Models

2.1 The Biopsychosocial Perspective

While the behavioral headache therapies employed today have emerged over the past 40 years, the view of headache as a psychophysiological disorder predates contemporary behavioral research. Notably, this view was advanced in the 1940s and 1950s by renowned neurologist and headache specialist Harold G. Wolff and his colleagues (Wolff, 1948; Simmons & Wolff, 1954) and influenced by Cannon's and Selye's work on stress and illness. The psychophysiological conceptualization was a critical departure from the prevailing "psychogenic" view espoused by psychoanalytic/psychosomatic medicine, which posited that headache arose as a result of emotional conflicts experienced in early childhood. Thanks to the efforts of Wolff and others, the psychosomatic formulation was supplanted by the contemporary conceptualization that more generalized physiological responses to stress contribute to a variety of psychophysiological symptoms. While Selye's (1936) early work defined stressors as physical events, Wolff offered a psychosocial formulation of the nature of stress (Simmons & Wolff, 1954). For over 25 years, Wolff vigorously pursued efforts to integrate knowledge from the social and medical sciences that would lead to better understanding of headache and other psychophysiological disorders. The work of Wolff and others reflected a major paradigm shift in medicine from a traditional mind–body dichotomy toward an integrative biopsychosocial perspective and was a precursor to the modern field of clinical behavioral medicine (Engel, 1977; Schwartz & Weiss, 1978).

Wolff is credited with articulating the once widely accepted concept of a "migraine personality," which he described as an array of personality features characteristic of migraineurs, including "feelings of insecurity with tension manifested as inflexibility, conscientiousness, meticulousness, perfectionism, and resentment" (Wolff, 1948, p. 348). Since Wolff's era, hundreds of studies have examined interrelationships between psychological factors and headache. His notions regarding a characteristic "migraine personality" have not withstood the test of time, and psychodynamic conceptualizations of migraine are now relegated to a historical footnote. Nevertheless, a strong biopsychosocial perspective of headache has emerged from those roots, with few headache clinicians or researchers prepared to dispute the significance of psychological, behavioral, and social factors in triggering and exacerbating headaches. This chapter focuses primarily on the behavioral conceptualization of headache within this biopsychosocial model, in which both head pain itself and resulting

A biopsychosocial conceptualization of headache has its roots in Harold Wolff's work from the mid-1900s suffering or disability are influenced by patient behaviors. For an overview of other approaches and the history of their application, the interested reader is referred to Rains, Penzien, McCrory, and Gray (2005).

2.2   Pathophysiology of Headache

Historically, the prevailing "vascular theory" of migraine held that the origin of migraine was the constriction and subsequent dilation of blood vessels supplying the head (Wolff, 1948). This once widely held view has since been discredited, owing largely to observations that vascular changes are commonly uncoupled from migraine pain, other attack symptoms, and response to treatment. The contemporary and prevailing "neurovascular" perspective now views migraine fundamentally as involving a hypersensitive CNS that is unable to appropriately modulate pain (Goadsby, Charbit, Andreou, Akerman, & Holland, 2009). Within this framework, vascular changes are phenomena secondary to primary neurological events within the brain. The neurovascular model attempts to account both for one's vulnerability to developing migraine and for the triggering of individual headache attacks.

Migraine runs in families

Vulnerability to developing migraine is partly a function of genetic influences, and family and twin studies have shown that migraine (with and without aura) has a significant genetic basis (Wessman, Terwindt, Kaunisto, Palotie, & Ophoff, 2007). However, the genetic influences are complex and likely multifactorial, and at present the precise genes and polymorphisms underlying these common forms of migraine remain unknown. Vulnerability also arises from experiencing repeated headache attacks, which over time further sensitize the cortex and brainstem nuclei involved in pain modulation.

An individual headache attack occurs when an already-vulnerable individual encounters an internal or external stimulus (i.e., trigger) that initiates a series of complex neurological events involving brainstem activation, cortical spreading depression (CSD), and stimulation of the trigeminovascular system. Activation of brainstem regions, particularly the periaqueductal gray, is involved insofar as dysfunction of these regions interferes with descending modulation of pain (Goadsby et al., 2009; Goadsby, Lipton, & Ferrari, 2002). CSD involves a slowly spreading (2 to 6 mm/min) wave of neuronal inhibition that traverses from the back to the front of the cortex and is the recognized cause of migraine aura (Goadsby et al., 2002), although CSD may occur among individuals without aura. CSD occasions release of glutamate and other substances that presumably sensitize and activate the trigeminovascular system, underscoring the long-neglected role of the cortex in migraine (Maizels, Aurora, & Heinricher, 2012). Pain occurs once the nociceptive meningeal afferents of the ophthalmic division of the trigeminal nerve are activated, prompting release of neuropeptides, dilation of innervated meningeal blood vessels, and neurogenic inflammation (Pietrobon & Striessnig, 2003).

Over time, the central nervous system of a migraine sufferer becomes further sensitized to internal and external stimuli

These resulting inflammatory processes further sensitize peripheral nociceptors and, with repeated attacks, the brainstem and cortex also become sensitized. The resulting "central sensitization" confers additional vulnerability to future attacks, to headache chronification, and to cutaneous allodynia (during or outside of the headache attack), in which a usually nonpainful stimulus to the skin is experienced as painful. Peripheral and central sensitization also help account for the neural hyperexcitability evident among some patients days or hours prior to the headache attack itself (i.e., migraine "prodrome"), as well as the resulting cognitive difficulties and fatigue that many migraineurs experience during postattack recovery.

Although the neurovascular model represents a major advance from the vascular theory, no one has developed a coherent integration of the interactions among these major neurological events. Moreover, this model does not fully explain all known aspects of migraine such as the prominent role of stress and emotions as attack triggers, prodromal and interictal features, the bidirectional influence of psychiatric comorbidity, increasing psychiatric comorbidity with increasing headache frequency, or the efficacy of behavioral therapies (Maizels et al., 2012).

Most recently, Maizels and colleagues (2012) developed an expanded "neurolimbic" model of migraine, in which limbic system structures interact with the pain-modulating circuits in the brainstem. Unlike other models, this novel conceptualization better accounts for relevant emotional and psychosocial factors, such as those influencing the subjective expression of migraine, chronification of headache, psychiatric comorbidities, and efficacy of behavioral migraine treatments.

As with the vascular theory of migraine, the "musculoskeletal theory" of TTH, in which TTH was viewed as resulting primarily from sustained contraction of the muscles of the head and neck, has been discredited. The pathophysiology of TTH is also complex and is now believed to involve a broader dysfunction of the CNS affected by both biological and environmental factors, although its underlying mechanisms are not as well understood as those involved in migraine.

2.3   Stress-Arousal Headache

Behavioral approaches to headache assume that interactions between individual and environmental factors play important roles in triggering and maintaining headache. The model is based on decades of research supporting the key role of behavioral and environmental stressors in inducing physiological changes/sympathetic nervous system arousal that, in turn, trigger headache

The stress-arousal-headache model is central to the rationale for behavioral therapies

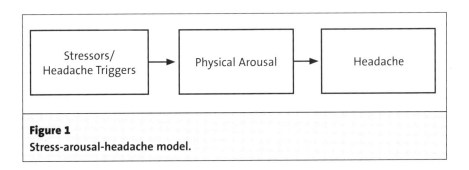

Figure 1
Stress-arousal-headache model.

among susceptible individuals (Penzien & Rains, 2005). Figure 1 depicts the relationship between stress, resulting physiological arousal, and headache in its simplest form. This schematic is useful for communicating to patients the key elements of the behavioral model in a way that is easy to understand and remember (see Figure 1).

2.3.1   Stress

Stress represents an imbalance between a demand and the resources available to meet this demand (Selye, 1936; Simmons & Wolff, 1954). Stated differently, stress is any challenge to the individual that may be perceived to be either threatening (e.g., an argument with an important person) or positive (e.g., an upcoming wedding). The stressful stimulus can be emotional (e.g., anger at standing in line), cognitive (e.g., playing a game of chess), or physical (e.g., exercise). By conceptualizing stress as any challenge, patients can enhance their awareness of environmental stimuli, thus elucidating targets of treatment that they might not otherwise have identified.

Stress affects headache in direct and indirect ways

Stress is the single most common trigger reported among headache patients, with nearly four out of five migraineurs reporting stress as a trigger of their attacks (Kelman, 2007). In addition to its direct effects of increasing physiological arousal, stress affects headache indirectly by contributing to maladaptive self-regulatory behavior patterns (e.g., poor eating habits, insufficient or excessive sleep, inadequate exercise, and smoking). For instance, a patient may be more likely to miss a meal or eat poorly during a time of high stress (e.g., working late to meet an important deadline). Stress also exerts negative effects on psychopathology, coping, and cognitive appraisals of pain; alterations in any of these factors can trigger or exacerbate headache.

2.3.2   Arousal

Stress-produced physiological arousal varies from minor sympathetic activation to a full-blown fight-or-flight reaction. The resulting arousal can affect nearly every bodily system, including the musculoskeletal (e.g., clenching teeth), endocrine (e.g., cortisol release), cardiovascular (e.g., increased heart rate and blood pressure), nervous (e.g., feeling dizzy or experiencing feelings of unreality), and gastrointestinal (e.g., stomach upset) systems. Some headache patients are readily able to detect stress-related physiological changes, but many have difficulty recognizing the more subtle physiological effects of stress.

At a physiological level, chronic stress prolongs activation of nociceptors, over time promoting central sensitization, such that headache patients under chronic stress may develop allodynia and hyperalgesia (i.e., a heightened response to painful stimuli), as well as delayed recovery from pain (Houle & Nash, 2008). The pain perception system, involving the periaqueductal gray and both serotonergic and noradrenergic neurons, interacts also with the limbic system, influencing both pain perception and response to stress, such that chronic stress prolongs activation and hypersensitivity of these systems as well (Maizels et al., 2012). It is likely that other direct and indirect mechanisms are involved in how stress-related arousal triggers individual headache attacks, although the precise pathways remain largely unclear. For instance, glucose metabolism is affected by sympathetic nervous system activation, and the resulting variability in blood glucose may sensitize nociceptors in the meninges and occasion headache through resulting inflammatory processes.

2.3.3 Headache

The natural physiological reactions to stress tend to be adaptive in the short term, enhancing one's ability to meet and overcome situational demands. Among susceptible individuals, however, these reactions place them at increased risk for headache onset and progression. Those experiencing chronic stress are likely to be particularly vulnerable to stress-related headaches. Moreover, experiencing recurrent headache itself is a stressor, which can further increase arousal and beget a self-perpetuating cycle of stress, arousal, and pain. Headache triggered by stress may be immediate or delayed by as much as a day or two, in which cases the delay may be influenced in part by interactions with other headache triggers. (Interactions between triggers and intraindividual variables render headache activity particular suitable to analysis using time-series research designs; Houle, Remble, & Houle, 2005). Headaches occurring during a period of relaxation after recent stress are colloquially referred to as "let-down headaches" and often may not be recognized by the patient as being stress-related. The physiological underpinnings of these temporal delays are not well understood, but clarifying the connections between stress, physiological arousal, and headaches helps patients appreciate and accept the rationale for behavioral headache treatments.

2.4 Contemporary Behavioral Models

The treatment program described in this book is based on a behavioral theoretical approach with decades of empirical support (Penzien, Rains, Lipchik, & Creer, 2004; Rains et al., 2005). Behavioral models of headache conceptualize headache as a chronic medical condition that is fundamentally a disorder of the CNS but strongly influenced by behavioral factors (Rains et al., 2005). The central underlying assumption is that headache sufferers can learn ways of behaving that can positively influence both symptoms and functional capacity. In this regard, the goals of behavioral treatments are to reduce headache frequency and the impact of headache on patients' lives by targeting headache-triggering and headache-maintaining behaviors. As behaviors are given paramount importance, teaching the patient specific skills to monitor and control stress and arousal are core components of treatment, along with attention to sleep schedules, exercise, and dietary patterns. To the extent that cognitions are of interest, targets of treatment are those related to controllability of headache, how stress is perceived, and one's ability to engage in adaptive coping behaviors.

Behavioral therapies emphasize development of skills to address stress and arousal

The behavioral self-management model has a broad reach, in that its core principles apply to individuals with significant health conditions and common comorbidities, as well as to otherwise healthy individuals wishing to learn ways to manage stress and other relevant psychosocial factors (Penzien et al., 2004). The model is applicable to the young and the old, across ethnicities, and to those with or without established headache histories.

2.4.1   Avoidance

Avoidance is a coping strategy commonly used to reduce anxiety or prevent the occurrence of a feared outcome. Despite its well-documented negative effects in other pain conditions, the role of avoidance in headache is only beginning to be explored scientifically. Historically, headache patients have been advised to avoid exposure to perceived headache triggers that are controllable. Although some studies have suggested that avoiding particular triggers may actually increase sensitivity to these triggers over time (Martin & MacLeod, 2009), these findings have had limited influence on clinical practice.

Avoidance may have long-term negative effects

Other, broader forms of avoidance in headache have more widely accepted negative effects. When headache occurs frequently, patients may begin to avoid activities and stimuli that are unrelated to pain (e.g., leisure activities, time with family, the work environment, foods that do not actually trigger headache). For some, overusing acute medications at the first sign of any physiological arousal may function as an avoidance mechanism. Over time, these avoidance behaviors become so widespread that they contribute to depression and anxiety, limited social support and engagement, and physical deconditioning, all of which further complicate treatment. Behavioral headache therapies educate patients about the maladaptive effects of unwarranted avoidance behaviors and teach them to develop more active and effective coping strategies.

2.4.2   Headache-Related Cognitions

Cognitive processes influence headache perception and management and involve neural networks strongly interconnected to those that underlie headache pain itself (Nicholson et al., 2007). Headache-specific cognitions influence how the patient copes with pain, adheres to medication, and responds to treatment. LOC and SE are especially relevant to headache and headache-related disability. Our working assumption is that these cognitions change as a result of success with the behavioral interventions described in this volume (Holroyd et al., 1984), although some practitioners target them more directly using cognitive restructuring and other formal cognitive therapy techniques.

Locus of Control
Locus of control refers to the degree to which an individual perceives an event to be under personal control versus controlled by external factors. A headache sufferer with an internal LOC believes that she is the primary factor in controlling and managing her headaches. Patients who believe headache to be out of

their control either (1) attribute management of their headaches primarily to their physicians and medications (external–health care professionals LOC) or (2) see their headaches as completely outside of anyone's control and instead to be a function of fate/chance (external-chance LOC). Variability often exists in an individual's LOC as it relates to different phases of a headache attack, with some patients believing more strongly that onset of a headache is under their control, and others believing that management of an active headache is more personally controllable.

A high internal LOC is associated with better headache treatment outcomes (Hudzynski & Levenson, 1985) and lower headache-related disability than an external LOC (Scharff, Turk, & Marcus, 1995), as well as a preference for behavioral treatments. Conversely, patients with a low internal LOC are less likely to initiate effective behaviors to manage triggers, reduce pain, and minimize disability. An external–health care professionals LOC is associated with higher medication use and potential greater risk for MOH, and an external-chance LOC is associated with depression, increased disability, and poor adaptive coping (Martin et al., 1990).

> **A high internal LOC is associated with a positive response to treatment and reduced disability**

Self-Efficacy

Self-efficacy refers to an individual's belief that she can successfully engage in a course of action to produce a desired outcome (Bandura, 1997). SE is a construct of central importance within the headache literature (Nicholson et al., 2007), as patients with high SE believe that they are capable of managing modifiable triggers and value adherence to pharmacological and behavioral interventions. They also report lower levels of psychiatric symptomatology than individuals with lower SE (Martin, Holroyd, & Rokicki, 1993). Increases in SE correspond with decreases in headache frequency (Nicholson, Nash, & Andrasik, 2005).

SE has been recognized for 3 decades as a potent predictor of headache treatment response, stemming from studies showing that SE (but not physiological changes) mediated the positive effects of biofeedback treatments on headache outcomes (Holroyd et al., 1984; Rokicki et al., 1997). Although the mechanisms underlying the effects of SE on headache are incompletely understood, sympathetic influences are likely involved, as low SE is associated with increased autonomic arousal (Bandura, Cioffi, Taylor, & Brouillard, 1988). The role of SE in behavioral headache interventions is discussed in more detail later in in this work (see Sections 4.1.7 and 4.2.2).

> **Self-efficacy predicts and mediates response to treatment**

2.4.3   Coping Strategies

Coping is a dynamic process of employing behavioral and cognitive efforts to manage internal or external stressors. Lazarus and Folkman (1984) differentiated coping strategies as being either *problem-focused* or *emotion-focused*. Problem-focused coping involves direct action to address the stressor or change the demands of the situation, whereas emotion-focused coping involves indirect attempts to attend to the psychological consequences of the stressor (i.e., one's emotions or thoughts). Pain is a potent stressor, and individuals vary widely in their methods for coping with pain. Common strategies for coping with pain include pain reduction efforts, relaxation, distraction, redefinition, expressing emotions, seeking emotional support, and seeking spiritual comfort (Keefe et al., 1997). The effective implementation of these strategies is often associated with reduced psychological distress and pain-related disability (Keefe, Rumble, Scipio, Giordano, & Perri, 2004).

Behavioral therapies promote problem-focused coping

Most research supports the conclusion that headache sufferers commonly use problem avoidance, self-criticism, wishful thinking, and social withdrawal as coping strategies (Hassinger, Semenchuk, & O'Brien, 1999; Holm, Holroyd, Hursey, & Penzien, 1986; Holroyd, Lipchik, & Penzien, 1998). These emotion-focused coping strategies are typically associated with poorer outcomes than are problem-solving coping methods (Penzien, Rains, & Holroyd, 1993), likely because they do not directly address perceived stressors. For instance, avoidance and disengagement, two emotion-focused coping strategies, are associated with increased headache severity, vomiting, and nausea (Ford, Calhoun, Kahn, Mann, & Finkel, 2008). The behavioral self-management strategies outlined in this volume represent problem-focused skills designed to foster active coping.

2.5   Treatment Implications of the Model

Behavioral headache therapies aim to reduce both frequency of headache and headache-related disability during and between headache attacks. The principal targets of treatment are the individual's headache-related behaviors and physiological responses. Specifically, treatment aims to (1) identify behavioral risk factors for headache, (2) modify headache-related behaviors and cognitions, (3) identify and alter physiological arousal that can precipitate headache, (4) develop a comprehensive plan for managing potential headache triggers, and (5) optimize adherence to medications and behavioral change. In brief, the goal of treatment informed by a behavioral perspective is to foster a self-management approach to headache that empowers the patient to assume control over virtually all aspects of the headache experience. The self-management approach to chronic conditions emphasizes identification of realistic goals as informed through self-monitoring of disorder-related variables, functional analysis of behavioral antecedents and consequences, and enacting discrete behaviors to foster symptom and disability reduction and promote long-term SE for managing the condition (Penzien et al., 2004).

3

Diagnosis and Treatment Indications

3.1   Medical History and Headache Diagnosis

Although many headache patients who present for treatment to a mental health provider have already received a headache diagnosis from a physician, assessment of the patient's headache symptomatology is nonetheless required for all patients. Confirming a primary headache diagnosis of migraine or TTH is imperative insofar as the efficacy of behavioral interventions for other headache disorders is unproven. Identification of any of the red flags outlined previously (see Section 1.6) requires referral to a medical provider for evaluation, as do any self-referred patients who have not been evaluated by a physician within the past 2 years.

The diagnostic roles of the mental health provider are to establish a headache diagnosis by assessing core headache symptoms, refer for medical evaluation for medication management or to evaluate red flags, and to assess relevant psychological factors (e.g., disability, psychiatric comorbidities, stress, poor lifestyle habits, behavioral triggers, coping skills, cognitions). The principal roles of the physician are to assess the need for medical testing or pharmacotherapy and to prescribe and manage acute or prophylactic medications. Many physicians routinely see headache patients, but few are specialists in the field of headache medicine. Identifying a headache specialist nearby in the community is ideal for making referrals of complex patients and for consultation purposes. To this end, the American Headache Society's Committee for Headache Education maintains a website that both providers and patients can use to locate nearby professionals with expertise in headache (http://www.achenet.org). As with other chronic disorders, regular communication between a mental health provider and physician is essential for optimal integrative care.

Communication between mental health care providers and physicians is essential for optimal collaborative care

3.2   Assessment of the Headache Patient

3.2.1   Domains of Assessment

Headache Diagnosis and History
All headache patients who present for behavioral treatment should be administered a headache diagnostic interview, even if they have an established diagnosis from their referring provider. The diagnostic interview helps establish (or confirm) the diagnosis and rule out more refractory conditions that merit referral to a headache specialist, such as cluster headache, MOH, and PTHA.

Obtaining a Headache Baseline

Obtaining accurate information about baseline headache characteristics is essential prior to initiating treatment. To obtain the most accurate baseline, patients are asked to self-monitor their headaches daily for a minimum of 2 weeks, and ideally 4–5 weeks, after the intake and before the first treatment session. A 2-week self-monitoring period may be sufficient for patients who have a longstanding pattern of near-daily attacks. For all others, a 4–5 week baseline is recommended; inclusion of a fifth week for normally cycling women provides headache data during all phases of the menstrual cycle (Penzien et al., 2005).

Disability and Functional Impairment

Because improved adjustment to living with recurrent headache is a significant goal of treatment, headache-related disability should be assessed at intake and throughout treatment as a means of monitoring progress. The HIT-6 is an ideal tool for this purpose. The MIDAS may be a more useful measure for assessing disability among those with very frequent attacks (i.e., CM or CTTH patients) and over longer periods of time.

Psychological Factors

Functional assessment may help identify potential secondary gains

Efforts should be made during the intake interview to obtain an understanding of psychological factors related to the patient's headache presentation. These include current major stressors and stress management skills, unwarranted avoidance behaviors, perceptions of responsibility for headache management (e.g., LOC, SE), and social support. Sometimes, reporting of headache is maintained in part by reinforcing consequences from the social environment (e.g., a day off from school, reduced work or family obligations, attention and reassurance from significant others). In such instances, the provider should incorporate a functional assessment to identify antecedents and consequences that likely maintain this behavior. (Readers interested in functional assessment of headache should see Martin, 1993.)

Common Triggers

Retrospective reports often overestimate potency of potential headache triggers, necessitating prospective self-monitoring or experimentation

Headache triggers can be identified using data obtained from patient self-monitoring and by querying the patient directly about potential triggers. Particular attention should be given to the most common triggers of migraine: stress, menstruation, missing meals, and sleep disturbance. Bear in mind, however, that patient reports often overestimate the potency of potential triggers, as many patients selectively attend to or recall only instances wherein they experienced a headache after exposure to a potential trigger (i.e., often ignoring other times when exposure did not trigger a headache). The most accurate assessment of headache triggers occurs with prolonged self-monitoring of daily headache activity and purposely manipulating exposure versus nonexposure to a potential trigger, while holding other variables and potential triggers constant. More formal assessment and management of triggers is described in the section "Trigger Management Training" (see Section 4.1.5).

Comorbidities

Depression, anxiety, and insomnia symptoms should be assessed in every treatment-seeking headache patient, particularly those with frequent attacks who have been refractory to other treatments. The PHQ-9 and GAD-7 are suitable for initial screening of significant depression and anxiety symptomatology, respectively. Insomnia and other sleep disorders can be verbally screened for using the mnemonic R.E.S.T.: Restorative nature of sleep, Excessive daytime sleepiness, habitual Snoring, and adequacy of the patient's Total sleep time. Positive responses can be further explored by inquiring about typical sleep schedule (e.g., bedtime, wake time, napping habits, hours of sleep), time spent in bed awake, and other forms of daytime impairment (e.g., fatigue, trouble concentrating). Rains and Poceta (2006) provide further strategies for assessing and treating headache patients with comorbid sleep disorders.

R.E.S.T. is a useful mnemonic when screening for sleep disorders

3.2.2   Recommended Assessment Protocol

Table 8 outlines the recommended protocol for initial assessment of headache patients.

Table 8
Recommended Headache Assessment Protocol

Measure	Domain of assessment
Intake interview	History (social, medical, psychological), past/current treatment, psychological factors (avoidance, coping), headache triggers, relation with menstruation (for women)
SDIH-3	Headache symptoms/diagnosis
HIT-6 or MIDAS	Headache-related disability
HMSE-25	Headache management self-efficacy
PHQ-9	Depression
GAD-7	Anxiety
R.E.S.T. mnemonic	Insomnia
Headache self-monitoring for 2–5 weeks	Baseline headache activity

Note. GAD-7 = Generalized Anxiety Disorder seven-item scale; HIT-6 = Headache Impact Test; HMSE-25 = 25-item Headache Management Self-Efficacy Scale; MIDAS = Migraine Disability Assessment Questionnaire; PHQ-9 = nine-item depression module of the Patient Health Questionnaire; SDIH-3 = Structured Diagnostic Interview for Headache (3rd ed.).

3.3   Empirically Supported Treatments

Many interventions are available for treating the headache patient. Below we review efficacious pharmacotherapies as a preface to the behavioral therapies espoused in this volume, as these two intervention types are often used in conjunction and produce superior outcomes to either drug therapy or psychotherapy alone, for both migraine (Holroyd et al., 2010) and CTTH (Holroyd et al., 2001).

Readers interested in reviews of interventional medical procedures such as nerve blocks, neurostimulation, and botulinum toxin injections should consult Ashkenazi, Levin, and Dodick (2008). Although nonpharmacological options other than behavioral therapies exist for treating migraine and TTH, the behavioral therapies for headache included in this volume are distinguished by their strong base of efficacy research from decades of controlled clinical trials. Readers interested in the emerging but methodologically limited literatures on nonpharmacological interventions such as acupuncture (Linde et al., 2009a, 2009b) and noninvasive physical treatments (Brønfort et al., 2009) should consult the cited Cochrane reviews on these topics.

> **Behavioral therapies outlined in this volume are distinguished from other nonpharmacological approaches by their strong evidence base**

3.3.1   Pharmacotherapy

> **Acute and abortive medications are taken as needed for symptomatic relief; preventive medications are taken regularly to prevent future headache attacks**

Medications used for treating headache can be broadly grouped into two classes: those that confer symptomatic relief of current pain (acute medications) and those designed to prevent occurrence of future attacks (preventive or prophylactic medications). Acute agents are taken on an "as-needed" basis and are designed to reduce or eliminate current pain. Some function to interrupt a developing migraine before pain becomes severe ("abortive" acute agents). Preventive headache medications are those taken, typically on a daily basis, to reduce the occurrence of future headache attacks. They are prescribed to migraine and CTTH patients with multiple attacks per month, who have not responded well to acute medications, or for whom overuse of acute agents is of concern.

Acute Medications

General principles of acute medication management include educating the patient about how to use a particular medication, treating the attack as early as possible, avoiding use of acute agents on more than 2 days per week, and stratifying treatment initially as a function of headache-related disability and symptoms. Migraine-specific agents (e.g., triptans, dihydroergotamine [DHE], ergotamine) are recommended for patients with moderate or severe migraine or for those who have not responded well to nonsteroidal antiinflammatory drugs (NSAIDs) or combination analgesics (Silberstein, 2000). For patients with significant nausea or vomiting, a nonoral method of administration should be considered.

Table 9 outlines the evidence-based guidelines for acute migraine management as produced by the US Headache Consortium in 2000 (Matchar et al., 2000). At the time of this writing, the acute treatment guidelines are being revised, although major changes are not anticipated. The agents most commonly prescribed for acute purposes are the migraine-specific triptans and various nonspecific analgesics. Triptans ($5HT_{1B/1D}$ receptor agonists) represent the major pharmacological breakthrough in migraine over the last 20 years, the first-released and most commonly prescribed of which is sumatriptan (Smitherman et al., 2013). Combination agents (e.g., sumatriptan plus naproxen sodium) and alternative delivery systems (e.g., intranasal sprays,

Table 9
Summary of Evidence-Based Guidelines for Acute Drug Treatment of Migraine

Migraine-specific agents

Triptans[a]	Strong evidence: naratriptan[b], rizatriptan[b], sumatriptan[b], zolmitriptan[b] Other FDA-approved triptans include frovatriptan, eletriptan, almotriptan, and sumatriptan plus naproxen sodium. These agents were developed after the publication of the 2000 guidelines.
Ergot Alkaloids and derivatives	Strong evidence: dihydroergotamine (DHE)[b] Moderate evidence: ergotamine + caffeine + pentobarbital + belladonna Inconsistent evidence: ergotamine, ergotamine plus caffeine[b]

Nonspecific agents

NSAIDs and non-opioid analgesics	Strong evidence: aspirin, ibuprofen[c], naproxen sodium Moderate evidence: diclofenac potassium (oral solution)[a], flurbiprofen, naproxen, ketorolac IM
Combination analgesics	Strong evidence: acetaminophen + aspirin + caffeine[c]
Opioid analgesics	Strong evidence: butorphanol IN, prochlorperazine IV Moderate evidence: acetaminophen + codeine, butorphanol IM, meperedine IM/IV, methadone IM, prochlorperazine IM/PR
Barbiturate hypnotics	Moderate evidence: butalbital + aspirin + caffeine + codeine Inconsistent evidence: butalbital + aspirin + caffeine
Antiemetics	Moderate evidence: chlorpromazine IV/IM, metoclopramide IV Inconsistent evidence: metoclopramide IM/PR
Other medications	Moderate evidence: isometheptene compound, lidocaine IN Insufficient evidence: dexamethasone IV, hydrocortisone IV *Medications established as statistically or clinically ineffective (failed efficacy vs. placebo)*: acetaminophen, chlorpromazine IM, granisetron IV, lidocaine IV

Notes. Strong evidence: Proven, pronounced statistical (at least 2 double-blind, placebo-controlled studies) and clinical (clinical impression of effect) benefit. *Moderate evidence:* Moderate statistical (1 double-blind, placebo-controlled study) and clinical benefit. *Inconsistent evidence*: Statistically but not clinically proven, or vice versa. *Insufficient evidence:* Statistical and clinical benefits unknown. Route of administration is by mouth (PO) unless indicated otherwise (but see footnote for triptans): IN = intranasal; IV = intravenous; IM = intramuscular; PR = suppository.
[a]FDA-approved for migraine (in adults). Rizatriptan is FDA-approved for children ages 6–17, and almotriptan is FDA-approved for adolescents ages 12–17.
[b]Mode of delivery varies by triptan.
[c]Excedrin Migraine (aspirin + acetaminophen + caffeine), Advil Migraine (ibuprofen), and Motrin Migraine Pain (ibuprofen) are over-the-counter medications with FDA approval for acute treatment of migraine attacks in adults.
Based on Matchar et al., 2000. As summarized also in Silberstein, 2000.

sublingual tablets, transdermal patches, needle-free subcutaneous delivery) are now available. The triptans are to be taken as soon as headache onset occurs. Many patients do not experience optimal satisfaction with triptans because of high cost or side effects (fatigue, dizziness, nausea, paresthesia), or because they do not administer the medication early enough in the headache episode for optimal efficacy.

Efficacious analgesic medications include opioid analgesics as well as simple nonopioid analgesics, NSAIDs, and combination analgesics (acetaminophen plus aspirin plus caffeine), any of which may lead to MOH if used more than 2–3 days per week.

Preventive Medications

Identifying a suitable preventive medication often requires weeks of continued therapy to assess treatment response. In general, preventive medications are started at a low dose and gradually titrated up as needed, with attention to side effect tolerability. Table 10 lists the common efficacious medications as outlined in the most recent evidence-based guidelines from the American Academy of Neurology and the American Headache Society (Holland et al., 2012; Silberstein et al., 2012). Medications most commonly prescribed for migraine prophylaxis are the tricyclic antidepressants, antiepileptics, and beta-blockers, although various agents from other classes have shown some evidence of efficacy (see Table 10).

Table 10
Summary of Evidence-Based Guidelines for Preventive[a] Drug Treatment of Migraine

Angiotensin receptor blockers and angiotensin-converting enzyme (ACE) inhibitors	Weak evidence: candesartan, lisinopril
Alpha agonists	Weak evidence: clonidine, guanfacine
Antithrombotics	Insufficient evidence: acenocoumarol, coumadin
Antidepressants	Moderate evidence: amitriptyline, venlafaxine Insufficient evidence: fluoxetine, fluvoxamine, protriptyline
Antiepileptic drugs	Strong evidence: divalproex sodium[b], sodium valproate[b], topiramate[b] Weak evidence: carbamazepine *Clinical context: Treatment with these agents requires careful follow-up and testing because of teratogenicity risks, pancreatitis, liver failure, and weight gain.*
Beta-blockers	Strong evidence: metoprolol, propranolol[b], timolol[b] Moderate evidence: atenolol, nadolol Weak evidence: nebivolol, pindolol

Table 10 (continued)

Triptans (for short-term prevention of menstrually related migraine only)	Strong evidence: frovatriptan Moderate evidence: naratriptan, zolmitriptan
Histamines/antihistamines	Moderate evidence: histamine (subcutaneous) Weak evidence: cyproheptadine
Nonsteroidal antiinflammatory drugs (NSAIDs)	Moderate evidence: fenoprofen, ibuprofen, ketoprofen, naproxen, naproxen sodium Weak evidence: flurbiprofen, mefenamic acid *Clinical context: Regular or daily use of NSAIDs for the treatment of migraine can induce MOH.*
Herbal preparations, vitamins, minerals, and other interventions	Strong evidence: petasites (butterbur) Moderate evidence: riboflavin, magnesium, MIG-99 (feverfew) Weak evidence: Coenzyme Q10, estrogen

Medications established as not effective, probably ineffective, or possibly ineffective
Not effective: lamotrigine
Probably not effective: clomipramine
Possibly not effective: acebutolol, clonazepam, nabumetone, oxcarbazepine, telmisartan

Note. Strong evidence: Established as effective and should be offered for migraine prevention. *Moderate evidence:* Established as probably effective and should be considered for migraine prevention. *Weak evidence:* Established as possibly effective and may be considered for migraine prevention. *Insufficient evidence:* Evidence is conflicting or inadequate to support or refute use for migraine prevention.
[a]Prevention as measured by reduced migraine attack frequency, reduced number of migraine days, and/or reduced attack severity.
[b]FDA-approved for migraine (in adults). Topiramate has FDA approval for adolescents ages 12–17.
Adapted from Silberstein et al., 2012, and Holland et al., 2012.

Amitriptyline is efficacious as a headache preventive presumably because of its noradrenergic and serotonergic properties. Although the therapeutic dose for migraine is typically lower than that required for treating depression, amitriptyline's antihistaminic side effects of sedation and weight gain often limit tolerability. The SSRIs appear to be no more effective than placebo for the prevention of either migraine or CTTH (Moja, Cusi, Sterzi, & Canepari, 2005), and more rigorous trials are needed to evaluate the newer serotonin-norepinephrine reuptake inhibitors (SNRIs). Unlike many other antiepileptics, topiramate is commonly associated with modest weight loss, although it often produces significant cognitive side effects. Three of the triptans have efficacy for prevention of menstrually related migraine when used on a short-term basis 1–2 days prior to and several days during menstruation.

The SSRIs are not efficacious for migraine

Injection of botulinum toxin (Botox) has been approved by the FDA for the preventive treatment of CM only and commonly requires readministration every 3–6 months. This treatment remains controversial among headache profession-als because of its substantial cost, invasive nature, nonsuperiority to other established preventive medications, and modest clinical benefit compared with placebo (2 fewer migraine days/month; Jackson, Kuriyama, & Hayashino, 2012).

When Pharmacological Treatment Fails

Lipton and colleagues (2003) reviewed the most common reasons for medication treatment sometimes failing (see Table 11). Although individual differences in pharmacogenomic factors certainly affect one's response to medica-

Table 11
Why Headache Treatments Fail

Diagnosis is incomplete or incorrect
– Incorrect primary headache diagnosis
  • Migraine headache diagnosed as sinus or tension headache
  • Cluster headache diagnosed as migraine headache
– Secondary disorders unrecognized
  • High and low pressure headache syndromes
  • Chronic sinusitis or other sinus etiologies
  • Cervical disorders

Exacerbating factors have been overlooked
  • Medication overuse
  • Hormonal factors
  • Dietary factors
  • Lifestyle factors
  • Occupational/environmental factors

Inadequate pharmacotherapy
– Acute therapy
  • Lack of migraine-specific therapy
  • Delay of treatment during an attack
  • Failure to use combined therapy (triptan + antiinflammatory or antiemetic)
– Preventive therapy
  • Failure to titrate to therapeutic dose for adequate period of time
  • Hesitation to use rational polypharmacy
  • Patient nonadherence

Inadequate behavioral therapy

Comorbid disorders
– Other chronic pain disorders
– Psychiatric disorders

Adapted from Lipton, Silberstein, Saper, Bigal, & Goadsby, 2003.

Ignoring behavioral factors is a major contributor to treatment failure

tion, most other reasons for treatment failure are a function of patient and provider behaviors and thus amenable to change. In our experience, apart from MOH, the most common reason for failure of headache therapies is inadequate attention to behavioral variables such as exacerbating lifestyle factors, poor stress management skills, comorbid psychiatric disorders, and a belief that headache is out of the patient's control.

3.3.2   Behavioral Therapies

The primary components of virtually all well-established behavioral therapies for headache are training in (1) relaxation, (2) biofeedback, and (3)
stress management. Typically, two or even all three of these components are
administered in combination. Relaxation and biofeedback are commonly
designed to reduce physical arousal associated with headache. Stress management aims to reduce stress by teaching patients to recognize headache-
related stressors and develop more adaptive methods of coping. Education
and self-monitoring are integrated throughout each of these three major
interventions. Other treatment strategies include trigger management (i.e.,
learning to identify and better manage headache triggers) and facilitating
adherence to pharmacotherapy and required behavioral changes. Acceptance-
based techniques are also gaining support and may be particularly useful for
headache patients who have proven refractory to standard pharmacological
or behavioral interventions or to facilitate improvements in disability and
quality of life.

> Relaxation, biofeedback, and stress management are the core components of behavioral treatment

In traditional mental health settings, behavioral therapies for headache
are typically administered over the course of 8–12 weekly sessions. In many
outpatient medical settings, where time constraints do not typically allow
such frequent sessions, treatment is delivered in 3–5 biweekly or monthly sessions in conjunction with brief telephone check-ins to assess adherence and
progress. These sessions are often scheduled on the same day as the patient's
medication management visits. Both the standard and briefer approaches have
strong efficacy as discussed later (see Section 4.4.1).

3.4   Factors Influencing Treatment Decisions

3.4.1   Age

Young and middle-aged adults are often good candidates for behavioral interventions. A meta-analysis of results from 36 studies of patient and treatment
variables among individuals with recurrent TTH found that age was the strongest predictor of treatment outcome, accounting for 30% of outcome variance
(Holroyd & Penzien, 1986). Younger samples (mean ages 19–35) averaged a
55% reduction in headache, compared with a 34% reduction in samples with
mean ages 36–52.

Older age was thus associated with poorer outcomes when standard behavioral headache interventions were used, but older adults can respond well if the
protocol is modified to accommodate their unique needs, including addressing relevant cognitive or physical limitations (Blanchard, Andrasik, Evans,
& Hillhouse, 1985; Mosley, Grotheus, & Meeks, 1995). Older adults benefit
from allowing more time for initial skill development and from weekly phone
calls to assess progress and attend to potential barriers.

Children respond particularly well to biofeedback interventions (Trautmann,
Lackschewitz, & Kröner-Herwig, 2006), often obtaining even higher rates of
improvement than adults (Sarafino & Goehring, 2000). Pediatric patients

> Children respond particularly well to biofeedback interventions

typically have less complicated headache histories than adult patients, learn behavioral skills quickly, and often enjoy the training procedures.

3.4.2   Other Demographic Variables

Women and men both respond well to behavioral treatments for headache. Although ethnicity has rarely been studied as a predictor of treatment response, existing data and clinical experience suggest that it is not strongly associated with treatment outcomes (Heckman et al., 2009).

3.4.3   Education Level

The success of behavioral therapies depends, in large part, on the patient understanding the treatment rationale and being willing to practice learned skills outside of treatment sessions. Patients with low education level are likely suitable candidates for a trial of relaxation or biofeedback if they can practice these skills regularly, as these techniques are easiest to learn. Stress management training that focuses on cognitive-behavioral techniques, on the other hand, requires some metacognitive skills and thus can prove challenging for patients with low IQ or who have difficulty thinking abstractly. Patients with severe cognitive impairments are poor candidates for behavioral treatment.

3.4.4   Patient Preference

Many patients prefer behavioral therapies to medication due to concerns about medication side effects or cost. Individuals with a high internal LOC also prefer behavioral treatments, because these treatments emphasize self-management of headache. Patients with an explicit preference for these interventions are most likely to be invested in treatment and adhere to the treatment plan.

3.4.5   Headache Diagnosis

Behavioral interventions are most useful for patients with migraine or TTH

Behavioral headache interventions are not recommended as first-line treatments for patients with cluster headache, headache that never ends (i.e., unremitting), or headache attributable to secondary causes such as head injury, illness, or intracranial pathology. Behavioral treatments may be useful for improving coping and stress management among these patients, but their efficacy in reducing the frequency of these headaches is largely unknown.

3.4.6   Medication Overuse

Medication overuse will interfere with treatment until the patient is withdrawn from the overused medication

The likelihood of a positive response to preventive pharmacological or behavioral therapies is extremely low while a headache patient is overusing acute medications. Almost all individuals with MOH will need to be withdrawn from their overused medications to achieve success with other interventions. Patients with MOH or suspected MOH should be evaluated by a headache specialist or other physician who can initiate and supervise the process of withdrawal from overused medications prior to or during behavioral treatment.

3.4.7   Previous Treatment History

Patients who have not responded well to adequate trials of preventive pharmacotherapy may benefit from behavioral interventions, either alone or in combination with medication. Those with a prior history of nonadherence to other treatments (pharmacological or behavioral) are typically poor candidates for behavioral therapies, as they are unlikely to practice regularly the skills they learn. Commitment to treatment may be facilitated by having such patients agree to a 3–4 week (or 2–3 session) "trial" period of treatment, at which point continuing for the duration of the protocol can be revisited. Alternatively, a prior positive response to nonpharmacological interventions for other psychological or medical conditions is a positive prognostic factor.

3.4.8   Psychiatric Comorbidities

Data on treating headache patients with psychiatric comorbidities are scarce, though clinical wisdom suggests that these comorbid disorders portend a poorer prognosis for treatment. Some of these patients, particularly those with more severe psychiatric symptomatology, will also require interventions that specifically address their psychiatric comorbidity (Lipchik, Smitherman, Penzien, & Holroyd, 2006). Patients with personality disorders, those who are currently abusing substances, or patients with psychotic symptoms are typically poor candidates for standard behavioral headache interventions.

Patients with severe psychiatric symptomatology will likely require more intensive treatment

3.4.9   Hormonal Factors

The temporal relationship between a woman's menstrual cycle and migraine attacks is very relevant clinically. Women with pure menstrual migraine often benefit from hormonal headache prophylaxis, commonly non- or low-estrogen birth control preparations. (High-estrogen preparations can exacerbate migraine around the week of placebo pills.) Women with menstrually related migraine are suitable candidates for behavioral headache therapies, and even "pure" menstrual migraineurs can benefit from improving their headache-coping skills. Women who are pregnant, breastfeeding, or attempting to become pregnant often find behavioral therapies appealing because they pose no risk of side effects or harm to the developing fetus.

Behavioral therapies are safe for women who are pregnant or breastfeeding

3.4.10   Life Stress and Coping Skills

Because behavioral therapies for headache focus on improving skills for coping with stress, patients with high levels of life stress or with poor coping skills are appropriate therapy candidates, particularly for stress management training. Patients with multiple stress-related somatic symptoms (e.g., fatigue, muscle tension, sleep or concentration problems) often are well-suited for relaxation, biofeedback, and stress management.

3.4.11   Appropriate Candidates for Behavioral Therapies

The text box shows patient characteristics indicative of suitability for behavioral headache interventions.

Appropriate Candidates for Behavioral Headache Treatments

Migraine or CTTH patients with:
- Preference for nonmedication treatments
- Poor tolerance of medication treatment
- Inadequate response to preventive medication
- Medical contraindications for medication treatment
- Pregnancy, planned pregnancy, or nursing
- Significant life stress or deficient stress-coping skills
- High internal LOC beliefs
- Prior success with nonpharmacological interventions for headache or other conditions

---

3.5   Presenting the Rationale for Behavioral Treatment

Many patients referred for behavioral headache management are understandably unclear as to why their physician has referred them to a mental health provider. Others are skeptical that anything other than medication will offer much relief for what they view as a purely "medical" condition. Some will mistakenly believe that their referring provider is not taking them seriously or believes their headache disorder to be "all in their head." Many of these concerns can be allayed if the referring provider clearly explains the rationale for behavioral therapies at the time of making the referral.

Discussing stress and sleep provides a transition into more sensitive psychological topics

Most patients who are referred for behavioral interventions have very long-standing and complex headache presentations that have not responded well to other interventions, or they have personal reasons for pursuing nonmedication treatments (e.g., preference for behavioral therapies, contraindication for medication treatment). In our experience, brief education at the initial session is very useful for addressing patient fears and misconceptions. The role of the mental health provider should be clearly differentiated from the role of the referring physician. Patients concurrently taking headache medications should be informed that behavioral therapies are intended to supplement, not replace, medication treatments, and that combination therapy produces better outcomes than either treatment modality alone. In our experience, discussing the impact of stress, sleep, and behavioral triggers on the patient's headache provides a comfortable, nonthreatening transition to discussing more sensitive psychological topics (e.g., depression, anxiety, substance use, coping skills). Drawing parallels between headache self-management and the self-management skills involved with other chronic disorders that have strong behavioral influences (e.g., diabetes, asthma) is also helpful.

4

Treatment

This chapter outlines specific behavioral therapies used in migraine management. As described earlier, the common theme that underlies all behavioral interventions is patient self-management. A foundational principle of collaborative care is for the patient to actively manage her condition outside the clinician's office. This concept often comes as a surprise to headache patients who view their attacks as solely under the control of physicians and medications (external LOC) or who have not been instructed in self-management strategies. The patient is taught to view headache attacks as strongly influenced by behavioral factors, over which she has significant control. Of course, this message of responsibility must be balanced with not "blaming" the patient for her headaches. In this regard, emphasizing the interaction between genetic and environmental influences is helpful; patients cannot change their genes, but they can change or manage their environment. Treatment is designed to help the patient develop the requisite skills for managing headache and the belief that she can do so successfully.

Session Format

As with behavioral therapies for psychiatric disorders, sessions during behavior therapy for headache are highly structured and follow a prepared agenda. Within a traditional 50-min session, the majority of the time (approximately 30 min) focuses on teaching the patient how to apply a specific headache man-

Table 12
General Timeline for a Standard 50-Min Clinic Session

Content	Time allocation (min)
Review self-monitoring forms	5
Review any issues from at-home practice and application of previously learned skills	5
New headache management topic education and skill development	30
Develop at-home practice and application schedule for new and previously learned skills	5
Summarize and address any lingering questions	5

agement skill to her individual presentation. The initial 10 min are generally spent reviewing prior "homework" and recent progress, and the last 10 min focus on assigning new homework, problem solving around potential barriers, and summarizing the key concepts from the session (see Table 12). In cases where a 50-min session is not realistic, the session may be reduced to 30 min (5 min for homework/progress review, 20 min on skill development, and 5 min for assigning new homework/summarizing).

Structure and Number of Visits

Within traditional mental health settings, behavioral headache therapies are typically administered across eight weekly treatment sessions – that is, the length of treatment for headache is typically shorter than that for psychiatric disorders, which appeals to most patients and underscores the importance of patient self-management during and after treatment. The recommended treat-

Outline of Standard Behavioral Treatment Over 8 Weeks

Intake Assessment

(2–5 Weeks of Headache Self-Monitoring)

Treatment Session 1
  Treatment rationale and education about headache
  Progressive muscle relaxation (16 muscle groups)

Treatment Session 2
  Progressive muscle relaxation (16 muscle groups)
  Monitoring stressful situations
  Trigger management

Treatment Session 3
  Progressive muscle relaxation (7 muscle groups)
  Monitoring stressful situations
  Trigger management

Treatment Session 4
  Progressive muscle relaxation (4 muscle groups)
  Analyzing stressful situations

Treatment Session 5
  Progressive muscle relaxation (4 muscle groups, without prerecorded instructions)
  Problem-solving (SOLVE)
  Thermal biofeedback (optional)

Treatment Session 6
  Relaxation by recall
  Problem-solving (SOLVE)
  Thermal biofeedback (optional)

Treatment Session 7
  Cue-controlled relaxation
  Continued biofeedback training (optional)

Treatment Session 8
  Consolidation and rehearsal of skills
  Relapse prevention (targeting techniques for continued applications)

ment outline for administration over eight sessions is shown in the box. Most patients will benefit from at least six sessions, and others will require up to 12 sessions for maximal benefit. The course of treatment will often have to be longer for patients with complicated presentations, a history of being refractory to previous treatments, or significant psychiatric comorbidity.

In some cases, treatment may have to be abbreviated due to financial considerations (e.g., income, insurance, or reimbursement issues) or other practical reasons. In situations where a full course of treatment is not desirable or practical, do not provide a very small "dose" of each component from the full protocol, as doing so undermines skill development and generalization. Instead, two alternatives exist for abbreviating treatment: (1) Identify one to three relevant behavioral interventions that can be adequately covered in a few visits or (2) provide the patient with more training materials to read and apply outside of clinic visits (i.e., "limited-contact interventions"). In general, we recommend the latter approach as it has demonstrated efficacy and incorporates the full protocol but requires fewer clinic visits, thus placing even more responsibility for self-management on the patient. Limited-contact interventions for headache can be effective in as little as three to five clinic sessions as long as the home-based materials are supplemented with some type of brief contact with the therapist between clinic visits. These and other alterations to the standard format of treatment are discussed later (see Section 4.4).

4.1   Methods of Treatment

4.1.1   Health Behavior Education

Education is a foundation of behavioral headache therapies and without it, most patients will either drop out of treatment prematurely or respond insufficiently. Education is used principally to teach the patient how to view headache from a behavioral perspective.

Many headache patients do not have a thorough understanding of their own headache disorder

Advances in information technology have made it easy to access medical information, but patients should not be expected to separate reliable from unreliable sources, particularly those obtained from the Internet. Many medical offices provide high-quality information, but the information devoted to migraine and other headache disorders is often not as thorough as that on other common chronic medical conditions. Given the brevity of physician office visits, most headache patients will present for behavioral treatment with an incomplete understanding of their own headache condition. In addition to education about headache itself, health behavior education typically addresses the topics outlined below.

Reviewing the biopsychosocial model of headache is useful for helping the patient understand the relevance of behavioral factors

Role of Behavioral Factors

Many treatment-seeking patients, particularly those who are not self-referred, wonder how behavioral issues can be relevant, as migraine is a genetic, neurological disorder. Reviewing the biopsychosocial model and having the patient articulate ways in which her own behaviors, thoughts, and emotions have affected her headache helps highlight the value of self-management.

Begin with a discussion of the roles of stress, sleep, and missing meals. Each of these is a behavioral factor over which the patient can exert control and that influences headache activity; headache in turn produces changes in behaviors, thoughts, and emotions. This tactic is often less threatening than directly discussing other psychological issues or unintentionally implying that the patient's headaches are psychological in origin. The overarching theme is to help patients realize that they can exert some control over their headaches, rather than letting their pain control them.

Roles of Stress and Physiological Arousal on Headache

Many patients recognize that "stress" is a headache trigger but do not know why. They may wonder how stress management or relaxation can help. Reviewing the stress-arousal-headache connection helps patients realize which stages in this cycle the various behavioral interventions target. Stress management and trigger management aim to reduce stress and other precipitants of headache. Relaxation and biofeedback, on the other hand, target the physiological arousal that directly precedes many attacks.

The Structure of Behavioral Treatment

For many patients, this will be their first exposure to behavioral interventions for any condition. Give an overview of typical targets of treatment, outline the structure and length of sessions, and clarify your role (teaching, empowering) versus the patient's role (applying new knowledge and skills) in the treatment process. An additional point of emphasis is the importance of out-of-session work in applying the skills and techniques patients learn. Those who devote significant time to practice outside of clinic visits typically obtain the greatest benefits.

Frequent at-home practice is essential for optimal treatment success

Setting Realistic Outcome Goals

Educate the patient that this treatment will not likely be a "cure" for headaches. The ultimate goal is reduced frequency of, and disability from, headaches, and in turn, improved quality of life. Many headache patients view being pain-free as the only acceptable outcome of treatment, such that anything short of total absence of pain is viewed as a failure. Helping patients shift their expectations of success from being completely pain-free to having fewer headaches and being better able to function despite their pain can be extremely therapeutic itself, particularly for patients with CM or CTTH.

Complete freedom from head pain is usually an unrealistic (and often counter-therapeutic) treatment goal

A Word of Caution About Education

Education itself is not a strong predictor of behavior change and, as such, is most empowering when paired with teaching the patient a specific skill to which it applies. Relaxation, biofeedback, and stress management are the primary skills training approaches, and these components yield larger reductions in headache than education alone (Powers et al., 2013).

4.1.2 Relaxation Training

Relaxation training is central to all behavioral headache interventions. Nearly all patients can benefit from some form of relaxation as long as they take

Relaxation must be taught to the patient in a step-by-step fashion

time to learn and practice this skill outside of the treatment context. The most commonly used and empirically supported form of relaxation training is progressive muscle relaxation (PMR), a programmatic technique in which patients alternately tense and release various muscle groups throughout the body. Other forms of relaxation include autogenic training, mindfulness meditation, and deep breathing. The core components of all relaxation interventions involve providing an overview of the training procedures, teaching the techniques, facilitating regular home practice and self-monitoring, and refining application as patient skill improves. (Simply handing the patient a relaxation CD is *not* at all sufficient for therapeutic gain.) The focus here is on PMR, although other relaxation interventions are briefly described subsequently.

Patient Overview

Initially, the patient should be provided with a clear rationale for relaxation and an outline of the training procedures. A strong rationale is particularly important for patients who do not initially "buy into" the utility of relaxation for headache management. What follows is an example of a rationale for relaxation that can be provided to the patient:

> As we discussed earlier, physical changes in our bodies associated with stress and arousal can produce headaches. Oftentimes, people say they are relaxed but their body still has a lot of tension that they do not recognize. It is important for you to learn how to (1) prevent your body from becoming tense, (2) recognize when your body becomes tense, and (3) truly relax your body and get rid of that tension.
>
> Relaxation training will help you learn to control physical arousal and thus help prevent headaches. Research has shown that learning certain relaxation techniques leads to fewer and less intense headaches for most migraine and tension-type headache patients, so long as they regularly practice and use their skills. This relaxation training program is going to teach you a specific set of procedures – not just "trying to relax" on your own. You will learn to tense and then release various muscle groups throughout your body, step-by-step. By tensing your muscles first you can notice how different it feels to be truly relaxed. Over time you will be able to relax very quickly in almost any situation. Becoming skilled at relaxation will give you increased control over stress-related biological changes that cause headaches, and relaxation often produces many other benefits such as improvements in sleep and reductions in anxiety.

In addition to reductions in headache, relaxation often has other benefits

Linking the rationale for relaxation with the stress-arousal-headache model is essential, as is explicitly informing patients that successful outcomes depend on regular and frequent practice outside the clinic. Although relaxation training requires more effort from the patient than does taking medication, relaxation hardly ever produces any negative side effects. Informing patients that achieving a state of deep relaxation will be a positive experience improves adherence and instills optimism regarding the procedures. In addition to positive effects on physiological arousal, many patients report feeling less anxious, sleeping better, and having more control over their emotions. The opportunity to engage in pleasant imagery, focus on sensations incompatible with pain, and develop SE for headache management are additional benefits.

Some patients will report that they have tried relaxation before but it did them no good. In our experience, further queries almost always reveal that by "relaxation" they are referring to leisure activities they do for fun, use of an ineffective or unproven technique, or one that was not sufficiently taught or regularly practiced. In such instances, discussing what the patient previously tried provides an opportunity to clarify that what they will be learning is entirely different. Patients who have tried and failed a suitable trial of PMR (or who are physically unable to perform the exercises) may be able to achieve positive outcomes with another type of relaxation training (e.g., autogenic training, mindfulness meditation) or by instead devoting more treatment time to biofeedback and stress management.

Progressive Muscle Relaxation Training

PMR involves sequentially tensing and then relaxing the major groups of skeletal muscles throughout the body, while attending to the different feelings associated with being tense versus being relaxed. Relaxation induced by PMR is physiologically incompatible with stress as it reduces sympathetic nervous system arousal.

Traditionally, PMR, as developed by Jacobson (1938) and later refined by Bernstein and Borkovec (1973), begins by defining 16 specific muscle groups and teaching the patient how to tense, hold, and then release each muscle group in turn. Once patients become proficient with these 16 tension–release cycles, the number of muscle groups is gradually consolidated into fewer groups (seven muscle groups, then four muscle groups) until, ultimately, the patient is able to relax her entire body at once without first needing to produce muscle tension (i.e., "relaxation by recall").

> **PMR includes tensing and releasing a series of various muscle groups**

PMR is most useful in preventing headache episodes rather than aborting an attack that is well underway. Therefore, patients are encouraged not only to practice daily but also to use their relaxation skills as soon as they notice tension building or headache starting.

Clearly explain that PMR is a learned skill, and as with any new skill, regular practice is necessary to develop proficiency. As patients' skills improve, they will become more adept at noticing increased arousal and implementing relaxation. With frequent practice, some patients will notice improvement in headache in as little as a few days, although others will report little benefit from PMR during the first month of skill development. The maximum benefit of PMR often is not achieved until after 2 or 3 months of practice. Thus, alerting patients that it may take at least a couple weeks to develop familiarity with the procedures or to notice any beneficial effects helps promote adherence, particularly if positive results are not initially apparent.

> **PMR, like any other new skill, takes time to master; thus positive effects are often not apparent for several weeks**

Instructions

In the first PMR training session, physically demonstrate the tensing and release of each muscle group to the patient, and have her follow along so that any observed errors can be corrected. Audio recording the session or following along with a prerecorded PMR vignette provides the added benefit of having a recorded transcript to give the patient for home practice. Muscles should not be

> **Walk through the entire tensing–release cycle with the patient**

contracted to more than 75% of maximum and should be released if tensing produces discomfort. (Patients who are unable to perform a particular tense–release cycle are sometimes able to produce tension for that muscle group in a different way or, if not, may skip ahead to the next muscle group.) The following text box outlines a simple way to demonstrate PMR before initiating the entire sequence.

PMR Demonstration

- A muscle cannot be tensed and relaxed at the same time.
- PMR helps you to *become more aware of feeling tense and when you are feeling relaxed*. If you know that you feel tense, you can quickly take steps to relax.

Try an experiment:
1. Tense the muscles in your right hand and arm by making a tight fist and tightening your arm as if you were lifting something heavy (like moving a box full of books).
2. Keep your arm tense for 10 seconds. After 10 seconds, relax your arm totally all at once. (PAUSE) Notice how different your arm feels when it is tense compared with when it is relaxed. You may notice that it feels warm or heavy, as compared with before.

- If we measured the level of muscle tension in your arm immediately after you relaxed it, we would find that it is actually *lower* than it was before you tensed your arm. Over time, you will begin to notice how your body feels when it's tense versus relaxed.
- When you first practice this skill, you may feel awkward. That's not unusual, particularly if you have little experience practicing muscle relaxation. However, like most skills, over time you'll feel more comfortable as you practice.

Using verbal cues during PMR helps the patient remain focused on relaxing

Ask the patient to avoid unnecessary movements and speaking during the PMR exercise but to make minor adjustments in posture if needed to maintain comfort. After a tension–release cycle is completed, the patient should avoid moving or tensing those muscles again during the exercise. Instruct her to begin tensing a muscle only after you have provided a specific signal, such as the word "now" after the tensing instructions are read. For instance, the therapist might say, "By making a tight fist with your right hand, I'd like you to tense the muscles in your right forearm and hand *now*." Similarly, the patient should immediately and completely (not gradually) release the muscle tension upon receiving a verbal cue to relax (e.g., "OK, relax *now*). This method should be repeated for each muscle group.

The environment should be conducive to relaxing. Eyeglasses, heavy jackets, or tight clothing or accessories (e.g., shoes, watches, rings) should be removed prior to beginning PMR. Low-level white noise can be used to block out ambient noise. Answer any remaining questions, then instruct the patient to position herself comfortably in a chair with head and arms supported and arms and legs uncrossed. Lower the lights and instruct her to close her eyes, settle into the chair, and take several deep breaths.

PMR Procedure and Script

Immediately prior to beginning the PMR script, verbally assess the patient's current state of relaxation on a 0 to 10 scale (0 = extremely tense and not at all relaxed, and 10 = extremely relaxed). Relaxation ratings may be supplemented with, or replaced by, ratings of observable relaxation behaviors if desired or if the patient's ratings are of questionable validity (see Poppen, 1987, for detailed information regarding quantifying observable relaxation behaviors). Direct the patient's attention to the appropriate muscle group, instructing her to tense upon the preidentified cue. After tensing for 5–7 seconds, provide the relaxation cue so that the patient immediately and completely releases the muscle tension. Direct the patient's attention directly to the muscle group as it relaxes, instructing her to notice the difference between tension and relaxation. (This relaxation "patter" may be supplemented with suggestions of feeling "warmth," "heaviness," or "deep relaxation.") Continue with statements that focus attention on the feelings of relaxation (e.g., "Let all of the tension go. Continue noticing the difference between relaxation and tension. Focus on nothing but the pleasant feelings of deep and complete relaxation."). The patter should continue for approximately 15 seconds, after which the same muscle group is tensed for 5–7 more seconds and then relaxed again for 15 more seconds. After this 45–60 second cycle, proceed with instructions to tense the next muscle group.

> **Providing instructions to notice the difference between being relaxed and being tense helps patients learn PMR most quickly**

Example Script for an Individual Muscle Group

*By making a tight fist, I'd like you to tense the muscles of your right hand and fore-arm **now**. Feel the muscles pull, and hold the tension, noticing what it's like to feel tension in these muscles as they pull and remain hard and tight…. And **relax** … just let these muscles go (pause)….Notice how they feel now as compared with when they were tense before. Focus on these muscles as they continue to smooth out and relax more … and more … deeply … more and more completely … thinking about nothing but the pleasant, warm feelings of relaxation.* (adapt for each muscle group)

Lower your speech volume, tone, and rate throughout the exercise, par-ticularly during the relaxation portion of each muscle group. Be observant for signs of difficulty or tension such as slowly tensing or releasing muscles, grip-ping the chair or clinching teeth, crossing arms or legs, opening eyes, or mov-ing excessively. Once the entire cycle of muscle groups is completed, instruct the patient to scan her body to identify any remaining areas of tension and to repeat the cycle for a particular muscle group as needed. Table 13 outlines the muscle tensing–release instructions for 16, 7, and 4 muscle groups. The example script in the box above should be modified for each specific muscle group in the table (see Table 13).

> **Be attentive to the patient's nonverbal behavior during PMR**

After the last muscle group has been relaxed, begin to terminate the pro-cedure by informing the patient that you will soon begin to count backwards slowly from 4 to 1. On the count of 4, instruct her to begin moving her legs and feet, on the count of 3, her arms and hands, on the count of 2, her head and neck, and on the count of 1, to open her eyes feeling calm and refreshed. Have her sit quietly for 1–2 min and take several deep breaths to readjust to the environment. Obtain a postrelaxation rating (0–10 as before), ask her to describe how her body felt while relaxed, and tailor your patter in future ses-sions to include her provided descriptors. Ask the patient about difficulties and

Table 13
PMR Tension–Release Cycles by Muscle Group

Muscle groups	Muscles and instructions
16	1. **Right forearm and hand** (by making a tight fist with your right hand) 2. **Right upper arm** (by bending your right arm at the elbow and bringing your hand toward your right shoulder) 3. **Left forearm and hand** (by making a tight fist with your left hand) 4. **Left upper arm** (by bending your left arm at the elbow and bringing your hand toward your left shoulder) 5. **Forehead** (by lifting your eyebrows as high as possible) 6. **Upper cheeks and jaw** (by squinting your eyes and wrinkling up your nose) 7. **Lower face and jaw** (by clenching your teeth and pulling the corners of your mouth back in an exaggerated grin) 8. **Neck** (by pulling your chin toward your chest while keeping it from touching your chest) 9. **Back of neck** (by rotating your head backward and pressing it on the back of the chair) 10. **Shoulders** (by pulling your shoulder blades together and raising your shoulders) 11. **Back** (by arching your back and sticking out your chest and stomach) 12. **Stomach** (by taking in a deep breath and holding it, while making your stomach firm) 13. **Right upper leg** (by lifting your right leg slightly off the chair) 14. **Right calf and foot** (by extending your right leg and pointing your toes away from your head) 15. **Left upper leg** (by lifting your left leg slightly off the chair) 16. **Left calf and foot** (by extending your left leg and pointing your toes away from your head)
7	1. **Right hand, forearm, and upper arm** (by making a tight fist, bending your arm at the elbow, and bringing your hand toward your right shoulder) 2. **Left hand, forearm, and upper arm** (by making a tight fist, bending your arm at the elbow, and bringing your hand toward your left shoulder) 3. **Forehead, upper cheeks, lower face, and jaw** (by lifting your eyebrows as high as possible, squinting your eyes, wrinkling up your nose, clenching your teeth, and pulling the corners of your mouth back in an exaggerated grin) 4. **Front of neck** (by pulling your chin toward your chest while keeping it from touching your chest) 5. **Back of neck and shoulders** (by rotating your head backward and pressing your head on the back of the chair, while raising your shoulders) 6. **Back, chest, and stomach** (by taking in a deep breath and holding it, arching your back, and sticking out your chest and stomach) 7. **Upper legs, calves, and ankles** (by lifting both your legs slightly off the chair, extending your legs, and pointing your toes away from your head)

Table 13 (continued)

Muscle groups	Muscles and instructions
4	1. **Both hands and arms** (by making a tight fist with both hands, bending both arms at the elbow, and bringing your hands toward your shoulders) 2. **Face, neck, and shoulders** (by lifting your eyebrows as high as possible, squinting your eyes, wrinkling up your nose, clenching your teeth, and pulling the corners of your mouth back in an exaggerated grin, while at the same time pressing your head on the back of the chair and raising your shoulders) 3. **Back, chest, and stomach** (by taking in a deep breath and holding it, arching your back, and sticking out your chest and stomach) 4. **Both legs and feet** (by lifting both your legs slightly off the chair, extending both legs, and pointing your toes away from your head)

Note. Exercises within parentheses should be done by the patient simultaneously.
Adapted from Bernstein & Borkovec, 1973.

positive experiences, and remind her that achieving a state of extremely deep relaxation will require time and practice outside of the clinic.

Home Practice

At the end of the first PMR session, reiterate the importance of out-of-session practice. We initially instruct patients to practice PMR for 20–30 min twice a day, every day, and to self-monitor their daily practice using a Relaxation Practice Log (see Appendix 6). As noted earlier, providing a recorded PMR script on an audio CD or flash drive facilitates at-home practice. Help the patient identify times when there will be no interruptions, a comfortable chair (with head and arms supported if possible), and a quiet place without distracting lights or sounds. Problem solve around potential obstacles as needed.

Proficiency with PMR depends on frequent at-home practice

Relaxation by Recall

Once the patient becomes proficient with PMR using 16 muscle groups, move to seven muscle groups, and then to four. Most patients can learn each sequence in 1–2 weeks as long as they practice regularly, but the time allotted can be adjusted based on the treatment format used (standard vs. limited therapist contact) and speed of skill acquisition.

After the patient becomes skilled using four muscle groups, relaxation by recall can be introduced. Unlike the other three sequences, relaxation by recall does not involve tensing muscle groups. Instead, patients scan the first of the four muscle groups and release any identified tension by recalling the feeling of releasing tension from the earlier training sequences. This process is repeated until all remaining muscle groups are relaxed. The patient may repeat relaxation by recall once for any area(s) remaining tense after the first cycle. If after two attempts an area is still tense, the patient should initiate the actual tensing and release cycle for that muscle group. With practice, most patients can quickly achieve relaxation by recall in virtually any setting.

Relaxation by recall does not involve tensing muscles

Other Relaxation Training Approaches

Although PMR is the recommended and most empirically supported method of relaxation training for headache, some patients will be unable to succeed at PMR or may prefer another relaxation approach. In those instances, the following techniques are viable alternatives, although they do not always produce as deep states of relaxation as PMR.

Autogenic Training

Autogenic training involves imagining parts of the body feeling warm or heavy. Self-statements and visual imagery, such as imagining one's limbs feeling heavy, or of warm blood flowing from one's core to the fingers and toes, are used as cues for the patient to relax. Due to its relatively long history in treating headache, autogenic training is often the treatment-of-choice for patients who are unable to engage in PMR due to pain or other physical limitations.

Mindfulness Meditation

Mindfulness meditation is a vital part of Buddhist practice and has been used for a variety of health issues. Mindfulness meditation involves focusing one's attention on the present moment, allowing thoughts and images to come and go regardless of their content. Present-moment focus is typically promoted by instructing the patient to attend to her breathing, to simply notice the sensations of air moving in and out of the body, and to return to focus on the breath when distracted.

Deep Breathing

Diaphragmatic breathing may be useful for patients who have difficulty with PMR

Deep breathing (often referred to as abdominal or diaphragmatic breathing) is perhaps the easiest of all relaxation techniques to learn, making it a suitable choice for patients who do not have the time to learn PMR. Deep breathing can be used in virtually any setting to modulate arousal and is particularly useful for coping "in the moment" with stress. Surprisingly, many people do not understand that there is a "proper" way to breathe. When teaching deep breathing, at first the patient should endeavor simply to learn the technique correctly, but thereafter focus strictly on her breathing and relaxation and not on doing the exercise perfectly.

Inform the patient that breathing is relaxing when it comes from deep in the abdomen rather than the chest. Have her place her right hand flat on her stomach and her left hand across her chest. Instruct her to breathe at a normal rate, inhaling through the nose and exhaling through the mouth, such that only the hand on the stomach should rise and fall during each inhalation and exhalation, respectively. Learning is facilitated by modeling the technique and correcting patient attempts as needed; observe how her hands move and ensure that the shoulders drop during exhalations. Direct her attention to how cool the air feels during inhalations and the warmth of the air on exhalations. Once the patient learns how to breathe deeply, teach her to slow her rate of breathing by lengthening both inhalations and exhalations. Exhalations should be of longer duration than inhalations, and the patient should pause briefly before beginning to exhale. The target rate is 10–14 breaths/min. This rate is most readily achieved by silently counting each breath on the inhalation and thinking the word "relax" on the exhalation, restarting when reaching a count between 10 and 14. Once the patient becomes proficient at this skill, she can continue to practice without needing to use her hands.

Cue-Controlled Relaxation

Cue-controlled relaxation combines deep breathing and relaxing self-statements. As the patient practices deep breathing, she is encouraged to silently repeat "I am relaxed" during each breath: "I am" on the inhale and "relaxed" on the longer exhale. This allows both the breathing and self-statements to become cues for quickly producing a relaxed state in virtually any environment. Cue-controlled relaxation typically does not produce as pronounced a state of relaxation as PMR, although some PMR protocols include cue-controlled relaxation as the final sequence (after relaxation by recall).

4.1.3   Biofeedback Training

Of all of the behavioral headache interventions used for reducing arousal, biofeedback has perhaps the most name recognition. Biofeedback involves teaching patients how to self-regulate physiological responses presumed to be outside of voluntary control. Biofeedback instruments "feed back" real-time physiological data to the patient, which in sophisticated systems typically involves an audio tone or visual display that changes as the physiological response changes. Many headache patients believe that they have virtually no control over their bodies, and the resulting hopelessness and frustration often complicate treatment. Learning biofeedback helps them develop an internal LOC and enhanced SE as they come to realize they can exert control over their physiology.

Various forms of biofeedback are used for treating headache, the most common of which are thermal (i.e., hand warming) and electromyographic (EMG) biofeedback. (Blood-volume pulse biofeedback is also efficacious for migraine [Nestoriuc & Martin, 2007] but has not been as well-integrated into clinical settings as thermal or EMG biofeedback.) For migraine, thermal biofeedback is most frequently used, the goal of which is to have the patient reduce sympathetic arousal by increasing body temperature. EMG biofeedback focuses on teaching the patient to reduce headache-related muscle tension, typically that involving the frontalis, cervical, and/or trapezius muscles. EMG biofeedback has been used primarily for TTH but is also effective for migraine, although the focus in this volume will be on thermal biofeedback given its relative ease of implementation without requiring digital equipment. Readers interested in EMG biofeedback should consult Schwartz and Andrasik (2003).

Equipment used for thermal biofeedback includes inexpensive alcohol-based thermometers that can be taped to the index finger, inexpensive fingertip electronic thermometers, and either portable or office-based digital devices with a thermistor. The digital devices afford greater precision of measurement and engaging feedback interfaces and are thus ideal for initially teaching biofeedback in the clinic. Pediatric headache patients often prefer digital feedback interfaces that resemble video games. The alcohol-based thermometers are inexpensive (around US $1 each) and portable and thus ideal for at-home practice.

> Thermal (hand warming) and EMG biofeedback are most commonly used for headache patients

Before Using Biofeedback

Successful delivery of biofeedback requires a greater level of provider skill and knowledge of psychophysiology than relaxation training. As such, some prior experience in biofeedback or a closely related area is desirable. Alternatively, behaviorally trained providers may develop some proficiency with biofeedback by reading an authoritative text on the topic (e.g., *Biofeedback: A Practitioner's Guide*, 3rd ed. by Schwartz & Andrasik, 2003) and being supervised by an experienced biofeedback technician. Resources and biofeedback providers can be located via the Association for Applied Psychophysiology and Biofeedback (http://www.aapb.org), and certification is offered through the Biofeedback Certification International Alliance (http://www.bcia.org).

Patient Overview

The exact mechanisms underlying the efficacy of biofeedback for headache are not fully understood, but its positive effects appear to be more a function of patients' SE and perception of their ability to control headaches than the actual physiological changes (see Section 4.2 for a detailed discussion of therapeutic mechanisms). To avoid undermining treatment credibility, provide a rationale that biofeedback works through helping the patient gain increased awareness and control over autonomic functioning. By revisiting the stress-arousal-headache model, educate the patient that stress and sympathetic arousal cause blood vessels in the hands to narrow, and as a result the hands become cold (the origin of "cold, clammy hands"). When a person is relaxed and calm, the blood vessels dilate, and the hands become warm. Biofeedback training teaches patients not only how to identify these changes but how to take steps to actually increase their body temperature, in turn reducing the likelihood of headache resulting from sympathetic arousal.

Biofeedback helps patients gain control over processes related to their headaches

As with relaxation, biofeedback is more effective for preventing rather than aborting headache attacks and is best viewed as a technique to be learned over time with regular practice. Some patients are able to use hand warming to abort headaches during their very early stages, or at any time they become aware that their hands are cool. In our experience, patients understand and benefit most from biofeedback once they have first become proficient at relaxation, although biofeedback may be taught without or concurrently with relaxation.

Instructions and Procedure

Biofeedback training should be provided in a room with a comfortable ambient temperature (72 °F ± 2 °F, 22 °C ± 1 °C). Using one layer of porous or surgical tape so that the finger does not perspire excessively, help the patient attach the bulb of the alcohol-based thermometer onto the center of the fingerprint on her index finger. The bulb should be secure but not so tight as to impede blood flow. (The precise placement on the fingerprint is not critical but should be consistent each time.) After attaching the thermometer, have her sit quietly in a comfortable position for 5–10 min to allow her finger temperature to stabilize in order to obtain a valid baseline. Baseline temperatures are typically in the middle to upper 80 °F range (29–31 °C) but may range down into the low or middle 70 °F range (21–24 °C). The goal of training is to achieve a stable temperature in the low to middle 90 °F range (32–35 °C) for 5–10 min.

Target baseline and treatment temperatures are affected by both individual and environmental factors

(For patients with warm baseline temperatures in the high 80 °F or low 90 °F range [30–33 °C], an increase of just a few degrees is significant.)

Learning which strategy is effective in raising one's body temperature is largely a trial-and-error process. Instruct the patient to check the device only periodically to assess success, using this information to identify effective versus ineffective strategies. Remind her to be patient and to avoid trying to actively "force" a temperature change, but to instead adopt a more passive strategy in simply allowing hand warming to occur gradually. Each practice session should last no more than 15 or 20 min, because one's ability to maintain warm temperatures declines after this point.

Several strategies may be tried to facilitate hand warming. Invite the patient to experiment with multiple strategies from the list below to determine which ones work best for her. For some patients, a simultaneous combination of these strategies is most effective.

1. *Imagery.* Imagining pleasant scenes or images associated with warmth or calm (e.g., lying in the warm sand on a sunny beach, sunbathing by a pool, hands over a crackling fire, putting on a thick jacket, warm blood flowing to the fingertips). Imagery works best when the provider has a sense of what the patient finds relaxing before starting biofeedback.

2. *Autogenic phrases.* Silently repeating the words "warm" or "warmth" while closing the eyes and breathing deeply. Another option is to repeat longer phrases describing the hands and feet as relaxed and warm, heavy, and comfortable. Heaviness terminology may be preferred if the patient's finger temperature is cold and "warm" has not been successful.

3. *Deep breathing* (as described previously; see "Deep Breathing" in Section 4.1.2).

4. *PMR.* Patients proficient with PMR may employ relaxation by recall to assist in hand warming.

5. *Sensory focus.* Concentrating on and magnifying the physiological sensations associated with successful hand warming (even if the patient cannot describe the sensations).

6. *Music.* Listening to soft or soothing music with eyes closed.

7. *Mindfulness meditation* (as described previously; see "Mindfulness Meditation" in Section 4.1.2).

In settings using digital biofeedback equipment, the same strategies should be tried, but the patient should attend to the audio or visual feedback provided by the device to identify when she is successfully increasing finger temperature. Those strategies that result in positive feedback should be continued.

Home Practice

At the end of the first biofeedback session, discuss the experience with the patient and address any difficulties. Some patients will become frustrated because they desire immediate results; remind them that hand warming is not an easy skill to learn and emphasize the importance of regular home practice for skill development. We instruct patients to practice biofeedback twice each day for 15 min each time, in an environment with appropriate ambient temperature, comfortable seating, and without distractions. Problem solve around barriers to home practice. As with PMR, we assess biofeedback practice by

Thermal biofeedback works best when the patient adopts a passive attitude

A trial-and-error approach is useful for identifying strategies that work best for increasing hand temperature

having patients complete a Thermal Biofeedback Practice Log during each home practice (see Appendix 7). This log assesses starting and ending finger temperature, relaxation ratings, and duration of practice.

Most patients can begin to develop skill at hand warming in 2–4 weeks as long as they practice in clinic sessions and daily at home. However, as with PMR, the full benefits of biofeedback often are not evident until after 8 or more weeks of practice.

4.1.4   Stress Management Training

Stress management targets cognitive and affective responses to headache-related stressors

Unlike relaxation and biofeedback, stress management training directly targets the cognitive and affective components of headache. Because stress is a frequent precipitant of headache attacks for both migraine and TTH patients, stress management offers a face-valid introduction to behavioral headache interventions, even for those who view more traditional "psychological" treatments as stigmatizing. Although many providers and researchers use the terms *stress management* and *cognitive behavior therapy* (CBT) interchangeably, we prefer the *stress management* term because it is less stigmatizing to patients and because formal CBT techniques are not primary in many stress management interventions (including ours). Stress management is recommended for all patients but is essential for those who report significant life stress, have deficient coping skills, or identify stress as a significant headache trigger. The core components of stress management are providing a strong rationale, teaching the patient to self-monitor and analyze stressful situations, and implementing problem-solving skills to adaptively manage stressors.

Rationale for Stress Management

Patients should be provided with a nontechnical but scientifically based explanation for the relationship between stress and headache. Stress is the most commonly reported trigger of individual headache episodes among migraine and TTH patients. Stress influences the onset and progression of headache in multiple ways: Stress can provoke the onset of a headache disorder in an individual predisposed to the condition, trigger or intensify individual headache attacks, contribute to the progression from episodic to chronic headache, and increase disability independent of headache severity (Nash & Thebarge, 2006). Recurrent headache is itself a major physical and emotional stressor, leading to a vicious cycle in which pain and stress magnify each other.

Stress terminology has become part of the public lexicon for health and illness, and most patients have some familiarity with the body's physical and emotional reactions to acute stress. This surge of adrenaline is adaptive when the situation calls for an immediate fight-or-flight response but becomes maladaptive when it occurs continuously in reaction to chronic or frequent stressors. The prospect of gaining learned control over the body's innate stress response is almost universally appealing to headache patients, as it offers them benefits of headache reduction, improved quality of life, and diminished anxiety. Reminding patients of the stress-arousal-headache connection and collaboratively discussing one or two personal examples is usually sufficient to establish an adequate rationale.

Monitoring Stressful Situations

Self-monitoring enables patients to begin to recognize stressors and their psychophysiological impact. Stressful situations self-monitoring forms are assigned as homework during treatment. Patients identify stressful events that occur in their daily routines, at least one behavior/thought/feeling for each situation, and relevant outcomes including whether or not headache occurred. Encourage patients to provide detailed descriptions of their thoughts and feelings as they occur. Beginning early in treatment, patients should be instructed to record at least four stressful situations each week to gain proficiency in recognizing stressors and their responses. A recommended form for monitoring stressful situations is provided in Appendix 8.

Self-monitoring is a central component of stress management training

Analyzing Stressful Situations

Review assigned self-monitoring homework with patients at the beginning of subsequent clinic visits. Have the patient select the most salient and frequent stressors for analysis, especially situations she felt were not handled well or that resulted in significant distress. Ask her to describe her state of somatic arousal during the situation. Query for behaviors that were counterproductive or maladaptive and cognitions that were exaggerated, catastrophic, or self-critical. Pay particular attention to stressors that recur and that are associated with same- or next-day onset of headache.

Over time, patients will come to identify key venues and individuals that are frequent sources of stress, as well as thought processes that intensify emotional arousal and are associated with maladaptive behaviors. These stimuli often precede headache. In the example shown in Table 14, fear of public speaking in the workplace occasioned catastrophic thoughts, anxiety, and maladaptive behaviors (e.g., skipping meals) that put the patient at high risk for headache but provided therapeutic opportunities for problem solving (see Table 14).

Help the patient identify people and situations (i.e., themes) commonly associated with stress

Problem Solving (SOLVE)

The SOLVE tool provides a guide for teaching patients how to analyze individual stressors and formulate an effective stress management plan. The SOLVE Problems Worksheet (see Appendix 9) is used to help patients systematically learn and apply steps of problem solving. The steps are as follows:

The SOLVE tool is useful for helping patients learn how to better respond to and manage stressors

   *S*tate the problem
   *O*utline the problem
   *L*ist possible solutions
   *V*iew the consequences
   *E*xecute your solution

Have the patient **S**tate the problem objectively and rate the severity of the problem from 0 to 10 (0 = *not at all a problem,* and 10 = *very much a problem*). Next, **O**utline the problem with respect to what objectively occurred and how the patient responded initially. Many times, the stressor itself cannot be changed but the patient's behavioral response can be modified to yield a very different outcome. Brainstorm a **L**ist of all possible solutions, being creative to list even unconventional or unlikely possibilities. This freewheeling brainstorming process enriches the pool of solutions with creative potential options, freeing patients from programmed solutions, negative thinking, and helplessness.

Table 14
Self-Monitoring Stressful Situations: Example

Situation	Behaviors/thoughts/feelings	Result
(Describe the situation: what was happening, where it took place, who else was there)	(What were you doing, thinking, and feeling? Include at least 1 behavior, 1 thought, and 1 feeling)	(What was the outcome? How did you feel about it?)
Situation 1		
As soon as I arrived at the office today, I got a call from my boss. She told me that she was sick and I had to brief IT today on a presentation we had been working on for weeks, so that they could be ready by the Board meeting next week.	I frantically spent every minute until the 1:00 p.m. meeting rehearsing what I would say — I skipped lunch and didn't leave my desk for 4 hours. I was thinking "how unfair" "if she is sick next week and I have to present this to the Board of Directors." "I will look like a fool," and "I should call in sick." I was feeling angry and panicked. "Oh...#^*!?!?"	I actually knew the material pretty well, after weeks of prep. The presentation was over in 20 minutes. The group was complimentary of our work. I was relieved it was over. Maybe it was a good thing my boss trusted me to give the presentation. I almost made myself sick from not eating and went home with a headache.

Date: *11/11/13*

Day: *Monday*

Time: *8:30 a.m. – 1:30 p.m.*

Headache? *Y* N

Viewing the potential positive and negative consequences of each solution is the next step. Have the patient consider, for each listed solution, "What are the consequences, including pros and cons?" or "What would realistically follow if this solution were chosen?" Selecting a viable solution becomes a logical rather than an emotional process when patients rationally weigh pros and cons of alternatives. Executing a plan of action after anticipating potential barriers is the final step in implementing a successful stress management plan. Patients should be praised for working through the SOLVE algorithm even if an undesirable outcome occurs, as doing so will encourage them to continue using this method and produce improved outcomes over time.

Most patients are able to learn the SOLVE process in-session and identify at least one stressful situation in their daily lives to which it can be applied. The SOLVE tool can then be assigned as homework, and with practice, problem solving can become a model response to stress. Once the solution is executed, patients can re-rate the problem severity on the 0–10 point scale to assess the effectiveness of the employed solution.

Stress management is not a technique to be used in isolation. Most commonly, stress management is combined with relaxation or biofeedback training and trigger management. Relaxation, biofeedback, and trigger management skills thus may come to function as viable solutions that can be incorporated into the stress management (SOLVE) plan. Stress management training also helps identify individuals with psychiatric comorbidities who are candidates for more intensive therapy. When stress management is delivered in group settings, problem solving is facilitated because groups generate a broader array of potential solutions and provide emotional support for members.

> **Stress management is typically provided in conjunction with relaxation and/or biofeedback training**

4.1.5   Trigger Management Training

All headache patients should be counseled in basic healthy lifestyle recommendations including minimizing stress, practicing good sleep habits, and keeping a regular meal schedule. For patients whose presentation is compounded by numerous potential headache triggers, a more formal program of trigger management training is often indicated.

> **All headache patients should be counseled to minimize stress, practice good sleep habits, and maintain a regular eating schedule**

The goal of trigger management is to prevent headache episodes by implementing skills for coping with particular stimuli that beget headache. Headache trigger management first involves educating patients about common headache precipitants and teaching them to identify their own triggers through prospective self-monitoring and behavioral experimentation. Once associations between common triggers and headache are identified, patients learn how to apply behavior change strategies to modify their responses to triggers. Trigger management training can be carried out in the clinic with minimal cost to staff and patients, and many patients respond positively to trigger management training even if they are resistant to other behavioral interventions.

Well-constructed trigger management provides another means for incorporating self-management skills into patients' daily routines. Patients often gain awareness not only of individual triggers but also of interactions among their triggers (e.g., between stress and sleep, between stress and menstruation). As with other behavioral interventions, trigger management training provides patients with a sense of control over their headache attacks and enhances SE. Recognition of triggers also aids in the appropriate timing of taking acute medications.

Self-Monitoring of Triggers

Prospective self-monitoring with the Detailed Headache Self-Monitoring Form (see Appendix 1) is used to assess exposure to common triggers of headache: stress, menstruation, sleep, and missing meals. Patients should be advised that they may be especially vulnerable to headache during exposure to these stimuli and instructed to record them carefully during self-monitoring. Once the patient becomes proficient in monitoring these potential triggers, she may be encouraged to consider exposure to other variables encountered in the 24 hr prior to headache onset (e.g., weather changes, specific foods/drinks, any changes in routine, certain smells). Recording exposure to these triggers may be facilitated by customizing the detailed self-monitoring form. This may be accomplished by using written abbreviations for various triggers or by providing a checklist of potential triggers of relevance, assigning each trigger a number, and having the patient denote the time of exposure to these stimuli on the self-monitoring form (by writing in the number of the trigger in the grid).

Identifying Triggers

Regular review of self-monitoring forms allows one to empirically identify the frequency of headache onset or exacerbation within 24 hr of exposure to a potential trigger. Keep in mind that the effects of exposure to some triggers are not immediate (e.g., stress, sleep, particular foods), and that false positives are common. The triggers of paramount concern are those consistently associated with subsequent onset of headache.

Behavioral experiments are helpful for accurately identifying headache triggers

A second option for identifying triggers is to have the patient conduct a series of behavioral experiments in which she exposes herself to potential triggers only on randomly selected days, comparing over time headache outcomes on these days versus nonexposed days. For instance, a patient who suspects red wine triggers her migraine attacks could be instructed to drink a glass of red wine on different occasions and to refrain from drinking red wine on others, making a note of each time a headache results within 24 hr. In designing behavioral experiments, it is important the patient attempts to keep all other environmental variables similar (constant) during each trial and allows sufficient time to pass between trials to minimize carryover effects (see Turner, Smitherman, Martin, Penzien, & Houle, 2013).

Prioritize Triggers

Rather than asking patients to make a large number of lifestyle changes at once, have them prioritize the two to three most common or potent triggers identified from their self-monitoring or behavioral experimentation. Once patients become proficient in managing these triggers, they can work on applying their skills to other triggers.

Apply Self-Management Skills

As major triggers are identified and prioritized, patients are encouraged to apply self-management skills to address each trigger while continuing self-monitoring to assess the outcomes of their efforts.

For triggers that are avoidable, self-management involves limiting or eliminating exposure by modifying one's environment and behaviors (e.g., keeping a regular awake/sleep time, avoiding particular foods, dimming lights). The most commonly reported food triggers include aged cheeses, red wine, monosodium glutamate, nuts, caffeine, and chocolate. Most established food triggers, however, do not always result in headache, and although many patients will benefit from avoiding particular food triggers, most will gain far more from maintaining regular eating habits (i.e., not missing meals) rather than adopting an extreme "elimination diet" in which any potential food trigger is avoided at all costs (Rothrock, 2008).

Stress is not entirely avoidable but can be reduced by limiting exposure to common stressors, employing stress management, and using relaxation or biofeedback techniques. Women for whom menstruation is a trigger may be referred to a physician for consultation regarding potential benefits of low-dose hormonal contraceptives or prophylactic triptan treatment immediately prior to menstruation. Caffeine withdrawal induces headache for many individuals and can do so even among those who drink no more than one to two cups of coffee per day. Patients for whom caffeine withdrawal serves as a headache trigger often benefit from gradually eliminating caffeine from their diets (after being informed that a temporary worsening of headache for a few days is to be expected). For others, caffeine intake may induce headache. Patients for whom cigarette smoking is a trigger benefit from smoking cessation interventions.

Uncontrollable triggers such as changes in weather or atmospheric pressure cannot be easily managed, but patients can be taught how to predict and prepare for them to the extent possible.

Patients are taught to apply self-management skills to better manage relevant headache triggers

4.1.6 Acceptance-Based Techniques

Headache practitioners are beginning to apply acceptance and commitment therapy (ACT) and mindfulness-based interventions, paralleling a larger trend in chronic pain management. Traditional behavioral approaches to headache attempt to directly change physiological responses and headache-related behaviors. By comparison, ACT incorporates commitment strategies to change illness behavior and disability directly while allowing a more passive acceptance of pain and pain-related private events (e.g., cognitions, emotions). ACT views the patient's struggle to be pain-free as perpetuating pain, and instead attempts to help patients distance themselves from their pain-related thoughts and feelings (i.e., viewing them as merely thoughts rather than truths). In the ACT model, patients aim to reduce the suffering associated with these private events rather than alter their pain directly.

ACT employs acceptance and mindfulness strategies to "defuse" (i.e., distance) the patient from pain-related cognitions and feelings, as well as therapeutic strategies for enlisting commitment to behavior change. The ultimate goal is to increase the patient's "psychological flexibility," enabling her to make adaptive behavioral changes despite contradictory thoughts and feelings. Behavioral assignments in ACT often overlap with those used in traditional behavioral interventions and involve skills training, exposure to feared stimuli, shaping, and goal setting, but they also incorporate additional techniques such as experiential exercises, metaphors, perspective-taking activities, and an explicit focus on the patient's life values.

ACT shows promise in treating patients with headache disorders

To date, empirical evidence for ACT as an intervention for headache is limited but promising. Two recent small controlled trials investigated adding ACT to treatment-as-usual (TAU), one using eight group-administered ACT sessions for patients with migraine or TTH (Mo'tamedi, Rezaiemaram, & Tavallaie, 2012) and the other a day-long ACT plus migraine education workshop for migraineurs with comorbid depression (Dindo, Recober, Marchman, O'Hara, & Turvey, 2014; Dindo, Recober, Marchman, Turvey, O'Hara, 2012). Both studies found that ACT outperformed TAU in reducing headache-related disability and affective symptoms, even if pain itself did not improve or was not assessed as a primary outcome. At present insufficient evidence exists to recommend ACT as a first-line headache intervention, but practitioners may find these strategies useful as supplements to standard behavioral interventions, particularly for patients with significant disability, those who have very frequent headache attacks, or those who do not respond adequately to standard treatment.

4.1.7   Promoting Adherence to Pharmacotherapy and Other Interventions

Adherence is a potent moderator of the effectiveness of all pharmacological and psychological treatments. Adherence pertains to following through with medication regimens, keeping appointments, completing self-monitoring and homework exercises, and adhering to recommended behavior changes. A literature review by Rains, Lipchik, and Penzien (2006) highlighted the magnitude of nonadherence in headache care. In the case of appointment keeping, 40% of headache patients fail to return for recommended treatment after initial consultation, and an additional 24% subsequently drop out of treatment. Factors associated with early termination were concerns regarding fees, wait times, staff, insurance, and clinician's skills or character; changes in headache; and concerns pertaining to the treatment regimen.

Adherence to headache medication is relevant because misuse of medications can complicate headache and lead to MOH. According to the Rains, Lipchik et al. (2006) review, 11% of initial headache prescriptions go unfilled, typically due to cost, tolerability, and side effect profiles. Up to half of headache patients are nonadherent with preventive or acute medications such as triptans, most commonly due to adverse effects, safety concerns, or complex dosing regimens. A common phenomenon with acute medications is that patients wait too long in the headache episode before taking the medication, at which point efficacy of triptans is limited.

Nonadherence to pharmacological and behavioral headache interventions is a common problem

As such, *providers should anticipate that most headache patients will not fully adhere to treatment*. Concerns about medication side effects should be assessed in detail because patients are often reluctant to discuss these concerns; however, they can be anticipated and addressed at the time medication is prescribed. Other patients will have preconceived notions about pharmacological or behavioral treatments based on what they have read on the Internet, seen in the media, or heard from friends and family. Correcting misinformation and collaboratively negotiating, rather than dictating, the treatment plan will guard against these contributors to nonadherence. Because risk for nonadherence is fluid and motivations for treatment vary over time, patients engage in implicit cost-benefit analyses, weighing the benefits of adherence against perceived costs. Patients are only likely to take their medications appropriately when the perceived benefits outweigh perceived costs. For this reason, adherence remains important even when preventive medications are effective and headache has improved, because patients who improve may be less motivated by pain to take their daily medications, which can lead to relapse. Table 15 lists the major factors associated with treatment nonadherence. Adherence becomes poorer as the dosing regimen becomes more cumbersome and requires the patient to deviate from her routine (e.g., adherence increases on weekdays and decreases on weekends). Scheduling more frequent follow-up office visits improves adherence (see Table 15).

Some forms of nonadherence stem from inaccurate beliefs about treatment

As described in Rains, Penzien, and Lipchik (2006), a variety of strategies can be used to enhance adherence to treatment, such as modifying the clinic structure, objectively tracking adherence, simplifying dosing regimens, addressing psychiatric comorbidities, improving the patient–provider relationship, utilizing behavioral contracts, and enhancing patient SE. Formal strategies for facilitating adherence are warranted with patients who have been refractory to treatment.

Table 15
Risk Factors for Nonadherence

Treatment-regimen variables
Multiple medications
More frequent dosing
Dosing complexity (e.g., missing "window-of-opportunity" dosing with abortive medication)
High cost
Frequent or severe side effects

Psychological variables
Presence of psychiatric disorder (e.g., depression, anxiety, personality disorder)
Low self-efficacy
External locus of control

Social/interpersonal variables
Infrequent follow-up visits (adherence increases just before, and decreases after office visits)
Patient's poor comprehension of diagnosis
Poor therapy rationale provided by clinician
Patient's low confidence in therapy
Poor patient–provider communication/relationship
Lack of family or social support

Adapted from Rains, Lipchik, & Penzien, 2006.

Clinic Structure

Contacting patients to remind them about upcoming appointments or check-in on missed appointments is the most basic and cost-effective strategy for enhancing adherence to treatment. Strategies to increase appointment keeping include patient reminders (e.g., mailed appointment cards, telephone calls, text or e-mail messages), scheduling regular follow-up visits, and holding clinic orientations for new patients.

Tracking Adherence

Therapists are encouraged to adopt adherence facilitation strategies early in treatment and to assess nonadherence regularly, advising patients that adherence is a critical determinant of efficacy and will be assessed throughout treatment. At a minimum, providers should ask patients to bring medication containers to each session for review of pill counts and renewal dates as indicators of adherence. Self-reports and pill counts are less reliable than objective measures, however, and tend to overestimate actual use. Objective monitoring of adherence is facilitated by reviewing pharmacy refill records and by setting alerts in electronic medical records systems.

Self-reports of medication use often overestimate actual use

Reviewing self-monitoring of medication use or skills practice with the patient provides opportunities for positive feedback. Self-monitoring of headache medication use is indicated if the patient is suspected of not optimally adhering to acute or preventive headache medications (i.e., not taking medications as prescribed, taking acute medications too early or too late in the headache episode, or taking acute medications more than two times per week). The type of medication, time used in relation to headache onset, dosage, and concurrent pain severity should be recorded.

Adherence to Medication Regimens

Table 16 details strategies to facilitate adherence to pharmacotherapy, which should be employed after consulting with the prescribing physician.

Addressing Psychiatric Comorbidities

Comorbid depression and anxiety undermine adherence to a wide variety of treatments, reducing both the patient's ability and motivation to adhere. Routine screening and management of depression, anxiety, and insomnia are recommended as discussed earlier (see Section 3.2.1). Scheduling more frequent clinic visits, increasing visit length, and involving family members are also useful strategies for headache patients with comorbid psychiatric conditions.

Many strategies used in behavioral management of headache are similar to those used in behavioral treatment of psychiatric disorders

Many of the behavioral strategies for treating headache overlap substantially with those used in treating psychiatric disorders (e.g., education, self-monitoring, stress management, relaxation) and thus may benefit both conditions. In some instances, treating the psychiatric comorbidity directly may improve headache. For example, a brief behavioral intervention for insomnia demonstrated efficacy in reducing the frequency of chronic migraine (Calhoun & Ford, 2007). Readers interested in detailed behavioral approaches to addressing comorbid psychiatric disorders among headache patients should consult Lipchik et al. (2006) or Smitherman, Maizels, and Penzien (2008). Saper and Lake (2002) provide suggestions for managing headache patients with personality disorders.

Table 16
Strategies for Facilitating Adherence to Pharmacotherapy

Involve patient in decision making and plan
Collaborative alliance, negotiation, active listening
Elicit barriers (e.g., cost, side effects) and problem solve

Simplify medication regimen (via prescribing physician)
Minimize number of medications
Minimize dosing (once-a-day regimens optimize adherence)
Use fixed-dose combinations tailored to patient's headache pattern and lifestyle
Rehearse and role play decision making for more complex abortive regimens

Educate about medications and provide written medication/treatment plan
Acute vs. preventive medications
– Abortive acute medications (e.g., triptans): most effectively early in the epi-
  sode
  • Awareness of prodromal symptoms (including aura) enables patient to
    promptly engage in appropriate timing of abortive therapies or nondrug
    strategies such as relaxation
– Preventive medications: successful prevention is contingent on ongoing use of
  these medications even in the absence of headache

Consequences of medication overuse with acute/abortive medications
– Using these agents > 2 days/week can cause increase in headache frequency
– MOH makes the patient refractory to all interventions
– Acute analgesics associated with greatest risk for MOH
  • Narcotics have greatest risk for MOH
  • Then simple analgesic, sedatives, and hypnotics
  • But MOH can occur with triptans and over-the-counter analgesics
– Obtain list of all the patient's prescribed and over-the-counter medications
– Prescriber should set unambiguous limit for analgesic and abortive medica-
  tions (including over-the-counter medications such as aspirin and acetamino-
  phen)

Utilize stimulus control strategies
Link medication taking to regular activity (e.g., meals, bedtime, brushing teeth)
Cell phone applications and alarms, pill boxes, and other tools to cue medication
use

Note. The behavioral provider works to promote adherence to the prescribing physician's
medication instructions, consulting with and deferring to the prescriber for medication
changes. MOH = Medication Overuse Headache.
Based on Rains, Penzien, & Lipchik, 2006.

Many patients with psychiatric disorders benefit from combinations of
pharmacological and behavioral interventions. The SSRIs and SNRIs prescribed for depression and anxiety lack strong efficacy for migraine prevention
(Smitherman, Walters, Maizels, & Penzien, 2011), and other agents require
differing dosing schedules or titrations by condition that often prevent identifying one agent to simultaneously address both diagnoses. Headache patients
requiring complex multidrug combinations or with severe mental illness war-
rant referral to a psychiatrist.

Behavioral Contracts

Behavioral contracts help patients with significant adherence problems to take responsibility for their treatment-related behaviors

Patients who are frequently nonadherent or have a history of medication overuse often benefit from behavioral contracts, as do those who engage in behavioral patterns that threaten their well-being or the therapeutic relationship, such as patients with personality disorders or who engage in self-harm. These contracts, signed by patient and provider, clearly outline expectations of the patient's responsibilities and conditions required for continued treatment. Typically the contract includes an agreement to refrain from harmful behaviors and specification of unacceptable behaviors (e.g., cutting) versus acceptable means of conveying concerns or strong emotions (e.g., calling the provider's office). Behavioral contracts typically emphasize the patient's responsibility for keeping appointments, appropriate medication use (including the commitment not to obtain medications from alternate sources), and homework adherence, as well as consequences for failing to abide by the contract (possibly including discharge from the clinic).

Self-Efficacy

Numerous strategies may be employed to increase patient SE

Because SE is a potent determinant of behavior change, enhancing patient SE often improves adherence. SE can be augmented though a variety of strategies that draw on past successful experiences and build new skills through reinforcement of successively more complex adherence behaviors. Patients should first be queried about their confidence in self-monitoring headache, taking acute medications optimally, and in applying behavioral skills outside of the clinic. Behaviors for which the patient has low SE are subsequently targeted using one or more of the approaches below.

Verbal persuasion is the most common strategy for enhancing SE and stresses the importance of adherence, describes potential negative consequences of nonadherence, and provides reinforcement for performing desired behaviors. Verbal persuasion is most effective when the patient is asked to begin by making small initial changes that can be mastered to increase SE for larger changes. Supplementing persuasion with problem solving around potential barriers to adherence also improves its potency.

Performance accomplishment is a SE-enhancing strategy that has the patient perform the desired behavior in small, manageable steps and is often supplemented with recall of past successful experiences. Performance accomplishment is considered the most potent approach to the development of SE. By succeeding with smaller immediate tasks, patients develop a sense of competence for more difficult tasks. For instance, patients with low SE for taking acute medications can first become skilled at keeping the medication on hand, then in learning to identify prodromal symptoms, and ultimately in taking the medication upon first recognizing these symptoms.

SE for behavioral changes also can be enhanced through *modeling*, in which the therapist demonstrates the skill of interest in sufficient detail so that it can be duplicated by the patient. A patient's confidence in performing PMR or biofeedback, for instance, often increases after seeing the therapist perform the same behavior. For this reason, relaxation and biofeedback are demonstrated by the therapist when teaching the patient these skills. Group therapy settings often have individuals describe their own experiences or demonstrate particular skills using modeling.

4.2　　Mechanisms of Action

4.2.1　　Physiological Mechanisms

In the 1960s and 1970s, a combination of theoretical and technological advances in the emerging field of psychophysiology led to laboratory studies of the relationships between physiological and psychological processes, which, in turn, prompted exploration of clinical applications for physiological self-regulation (Shapiro & Schwartz, 1972). Around this time, studies appeared demonstrating that, through using operant biofeedback methods, individuals could develop a degree of voluntary regulation over physiological responses previously thought beyond conscious control, some of which positively affected migraine (raising skin temperature) and TTH (reducing EMG tension) (Budzynski & Stoyva, 1969; Sargent, Green, & Walters, 1972).

The rationale for the development of biofeedback, for instance, was derived from the widely accepted (but now discredited) premises that migraine was a vascular and TTH a musculoskeletal phenomenon. Accordingly, thermal and EMG biofeedback targeted supposed pathophysiologies of migraine and TTH, respectively. A more sophisticated understanding of headache pathophysiology and behavioral interventions prompted a reconceptualization of the presumed physiological mechanisms through which these interventions operated. The therapeutic mechanisms of biofeedback and other behavioral headache therapies are now recognized as being considerably more complex than simple self-regulation of physiological responses. This appreciation is attributable in large part to research designs employing false- or altered-contingency biofeedback control conditions (Rains & Penzien, 2005).

Behavioral interventions are not effective simply because they alter physiological responses

4.2.2　　Psychological Mechanisms

Andrasik and Holroyd (1980) employed altered-contingency biofeedback to evaluate whether self-regulation of muscle tension was the principal mechanism for the therapeutic gains observed with EMG biofeedback. Although all patients were led to believe they were learning to reduce frontal EMG activity, TTH sufferers actually were assigned to one of three groups: they received feedback that was contingent on (a) reductions in forehead EMG tension, (b) increases in forehead EMG tension, or (c) change in an irrelevant muscle group (forearm flexor). Irrespective of the actual feedback they received, patients in all three treatment groups showed similar and clinically meaningful reductions in headache at posttreatment and at a 3-year follow-up (Andrasik & Holroyd, 1983). Results from this and other altered-contingency designs (Cram, 1980; Phillips & Hunter, 1981) suggested that improvements in tension headache with EMG biofeedback training do not accrue simply as a function of reduction in muscle tension. These studies, among others, provided the impetus for reexamination and eventual discrediting of the "musculoskeletal hypothesis" of TTH.

Holroyd and colleagues (1984) extended the Andrasik and Holroyd (1980) study by also manipulating patients' perceptions of their success with biofeedback using a 2 (increase vs. decrease EMG activity) × 2 (high vs. moderate success) experimental design. As in their initial study, they found that headache improvement accrued with EMG biofeedback regardless of whether patients were taught to increase or decrease muscle tension. Importantly, greater headache reductions were reported by patients who received the high success feedback regardless of their biofeedback condition (increase vs. decrease EMG). Headache improvements did not correlate with EMG changes but instead with cognitive changes in SE and LOC. This seminal study was the first of many to demonstrate that gains observed with biofeedback were mediated by cognitive-attributional changes induced by behavioral self-management training, rather than principally via physiological self-regulation (Holroyd, 2002).

> **Psychological constructs predict behavioral treatment outcomes more than physiological changes do**

4.3   Efficacy and Prognosis

Behavioral treatments for migraine and TTH have accumulated substantial empirical support regarding their efficacy for adults as well as for children and adolescents (Rains et al., 2005; Trautmann et al., 2006).

4.3.1   Efficacy for Migraine

Since the earliest empirical report evaluating a behavioral intervention for headache appeared in 1969, over 300 studies evaluating behavioral treatments for migraine have been published. Virtually all of those studies have reported positive outcomes, leading many professional practice organizations to recommend use of behavioral headache treatments as first-line interventions for migraine, along with pharmacological treatments.

An authoritative meta-analysis of behavioral treatments for migraine by Goslin and colleagues (1999), supported by the Agency for Healthcare Research and Quality (formerly the Agency for Health Care Policy and Research), concluded that the various behavioral interventions for migraine yielded a 35% to 50% reduction in migraine frequency after treatment, compared with 5% and 10% reductions for no-treatment and for other control conditions, respectively (see Figure 2).

> **The US Headache Consortium guidelines concluded that behavioral therapies have Grade A evidence for migraine prevention**

This meta-analysis, consistent with other previous and subsequent empirical reviews of this literature (Holroyd & Penzien, 1990; Palermo et al., 2010; Rains et al., 2005; Trautmann et al., 2006), provided the basis for an evidence-based guideline for migraine management produced by the US Headache Consortium (Campbell, Penzien, & Wall, 2000). Member organizations of this consortium were the American Academy of Family Physicians, American Academy of Neurology, American Headache Society, American College of Emergency Physicians, American College of Physicians, American Osteopathic Association, and the National Headache Foundation. Focused on management of migraine by the primary care practitioner, the guideline for behavioral treatments is available online (http://www.americanheadachesociety.org/assets/1/7/04_HAConsortium_BehavioralGuideline2000.PDF), and a summary of the recommendations can be found in Silberstein (2000). The Consortium's

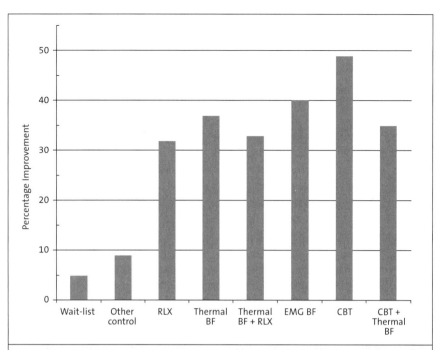

Figure 2
Meta-analysis of behavioral treatments for migraine. Bars depict the percentage reduction in headache frequency or headache index (composite of headache frequency, severity, and/or duration) from pretreatment to posttreatment. RLX = relaxation training; BF = biofeedback training; EMG = electromyographic; CBT = cognitive behavior therapy (i.e., stress management).
Based on Goslin et al., 1999.

principal recommendations regarding behavioral headache therapies (Campbell et al., 2000) are reprinted in Table 17.

Few studies have directly compared the efficacy of behavioral versus drug therapies for migraine. However, meta-analytic comparisons reveal behavioral interventions yield reductions in migraine frequency similar to both propranolol, an FDA-approved beta-blocker for migraine prevention, and flunarizine, an efficacious calcium channel blocker widely used in Canada and Europe (Davis, Holroyd, & Penzien, 1999; Holroyd & Penzien, 1990). Patients receiving propranolol, flunarizine, or behavioral interventions showed greater than a 50% improvement in migraine, whereas patients receiving medication placebos showed only a 12% improvement. While the two treatment modalities offer distinct advantages and disadvantages within particular patient subgroups, the best of the prophylactic medications and behavioral therapies are similarly viable for migraine management.

Behavioral treatments have similar efficacy to common medications used for migraine prevention

Importantly, a large-scale, randomized controlled trial (RCT) found that combining behavioral and pharmacological therapies for migraine (Holroyd et al., 2010) was associated with better outcomes than either treatment alone. In addition to receiving optimized acute medications, migraineurs in this study were assigned to receive (a) a beta-blocker (propranolol or nadolol), (b) placebo medication, (c) CBT plus beta-blocker, or (d) CBT plus placebo. CBT

Combining behavioral and medication treatments produce outcomes superior to either treatment alone

Table 17
US Headache Consortium Recommendations for Behavioral Therapies

Grade A evidence for migraine prevention	• Relaxation training • Thermal biofeedback combined with relaxation training • Electromyographic (EMG) feedback • Cognitive behavior therapy (CBT; i.e., stress management)
Grade B evidence for migraine prevention	• Behavioral therapy may be combined with preventive drug therapy to achieve added clinical improvement[a]

Notes. [a]This conclusion would now be considered Grade A evidence upon the publication of Holroyd et al. (2010) and Powers et al. (2013). Grade A: Multiple well-designed randomized clinical trials yielded a consistent pattern of findings; Grade B: Findings from randomized clinical trials were generally consistent but few in number.

included three to four clinic visits focused on PMR and stress management or thermal biofeedback, with at-home skills practice and periodic phone follow-ups. Only patients receiving CBT plus beta-blocker obtained significant reductions in migraine frequency compared with acute treatment plus placebo. Three quarters of patients (77%) in the combined-treatment group evidenced clinically significant improvements of ≥ 50% reductions in migraine frequency (vs. 34–40% in the other three treatment groups). Perhaps because they have differing mechanisms of action, combining behavioral and pharmacological migraine therapies clearly provides additional benefits.

Most recently, Powers and colleagues (2013) conducted an RCT to compare the efficacy of behavioral therapy plus amitriptyline with headache education plus amitriptyline among a large sample of youth with CM (ages 10–17; mean headache frequency = 21 days/month). Patients in each group attended 10 treatment sessions. Patients receiving behavioral therapy obtained significantly larger improvements in both headache frequency and headache-related disability than did those receiving headache education. Two thirds of those receiving behavioral therapy obtained a reduction in headache frequency of at least 50% (vs. 36% in the education group), which at 12-month follow-up had increased to 88% of patients. These data demonstrate the superiority of behavioral therapy to education alone and support its use as a primary intervention for children and adolescents with CM, a population for whom other evidence-based interventions are lacking.

4.3.2   Efficacy for Tension-Type Headache

Reductions in TTH frequency with behavioral interventions are similar to those seen in migraine

Closely paralleling the methodology and findings of the Goslin et al. (1999) review of migraine studies, an authoritative meta-analysis of behavioral treatments for TTH by McCrory, Penzien, Hasselblad, and Gray (2001) found that the various behavioral interventions for TTH yielded a 35% to 50% reduction in headache frequency after treatment, compared with a 2% reduction for no-

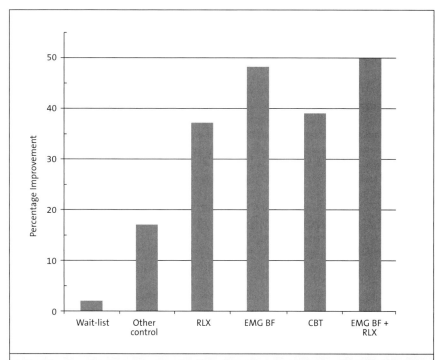

Figure 3
Meta-analysis of behavioral treatments for tension-type headache. Bars depict the percentage reduction in headache frequency or headache index (composite of headache frequency, severity, and/or duration) from pretreatment to posttreatment. RLX = relaxation training; BF = biofeedback training; EMG = electromyographic; CBT = cognitive behavior therapy (i.e., stress management). Based on McCrory, Penzien, Hasselblad, & Gray, 2001.

treatment and 15% for other controls (see Figure 3). The McCrory et al. meta-analysis is consistent with other past and subsequent empirical reviews of the TTH literature (Holroyd & Penzien, 1986; Nestoriuc et al., 2008; Palermo et al., 2010; Rains et al., 2005; Trautmann et al., 2006).

Holroyd and colleagues (2001) published an authoritative comparison of behavioral and pharmacological treatments for CTTH in which more than 200 patients were assigned to receive (a) a tricyclic antidepressant (amitriptyline or nortriptyline), (b) CBT (PMR and stress management), (c) combined antidepressant and CBT, or (d) pill placebo. Compared with placebo, medication and behavioral therapy produced larger reductions in headache activity, analgesic medication use, and headache-related disability, but medication yielded more rapid improvements in headache activity. Most importantly, a higher proportion of patients receiving combined therapy (64%) experienced a clinically significant reduction in headache compared with antidepressant medication alone (38%) or stress management training alone (35%). As with migraine, for CTTH each treatment strategy is effective when used alone, but better outcomes are achieved with a combined approach.

4.3.3   Maintenance of Treatment Gains Over Time

The effects of behavioral treatments are long-lasting

Considerable evidence indicates that among patients initially responsive to therapy, the effects of behavioral therapies endure well over time, with multiple studies showing maintenance of gains several years after treatment (Blanchard, 1992). For instance, Blanchard and colleagues (1987) found that 91% of migraineurs and 78% of TTH sufferers remained significantly improved 5 years after completing behavioral treatment.

4.4   Variations and Combinations of Methods

To address cost and access issues, headache researchers have devised and studied a variety of alternative intervention formats for delivery of behavioral treatments including, among others, limited-therapist-contact therapy, nonprofessionally administered therapy, self-help therapy, and Internet- or other mass-communications-based therapies (Rains et al., 2005). Each therapeutic approach examined to date has yielded successful outcomes and shown considerable promise.

4.4.1   Limited-Therapist-Contact Behavioral Therapies

The greatest empirical support for an alternative mode of service delivery has accumulated for the limited-therapist-contact or "home-based" behavioral treatment formats. Limited-contact therapy provides an efficient and economical mode of treatment delivery. In these interventions, headache self-management skills are introduced in face-to-face clinic sessions, but training principally occurs at home with the patient guided by printed and audiovisual materials (delivered via audio CD or the Internet). Consequently, only three to five clinic appointments may be needed when behavioral headache therapy is delivered via this format versus the 8-12 clinic sessions required for typical clinic-based formats. One or two telephone contacts, scheduled early in treatment, provide a means for assessing progress and adherence and addressing barriers to change. The following boxes outline the session structure for administering the traditional 8-week treatment program using either five or three in-office clinic visits.

Limited-contact behavioral therapies require only 3–5 clinic visits

Outline of Limited-Contact Treatment Over 8 Weeks (Administration in five clinic sessions)

Intake assessment

(2–5 weeks of headache self-monitoring)

Treatment Session 1 (beginning of Treatment Week 1)
  Treatment rationale and education about headache
  Progressive muscle relaxation (16 muscle groups)
  Monitoring stressful situations

Scheduled telephone contact (check-in regarding progress, adherence, barriers; End of Week 1)

Week 2 (no therapist contact)
 Progressive muscle relaxation (7 muscle groups)
 Monitoring stressful situations
 Trigger management

Treatment Session 2 (beginning of Week 3)
 Progressive muscle relaxation (4 muscle groups)
 Monitoring stressful situations
 Trigger management

Week 4 (no therapist contact)
 Progressive muscle relaxation (4 muscle groups, without prerecorded
 instructions)
 Analyzing stressful situations

Treatment Session 3 (beginning of Week 5)
 Relaxation by recall
 Cue-controlled relaxation
 Problem solving (SOLVE)

Week 6 (no therapist contact)
 Thermal biofeedback (optional)
 Relaxation by recall
 Cue-controlled relaxation
 Problem solving (SOLVE)

Treatment Session 4 (beginning of Week 7)
 Continued relaxation and biofeedback training
 Problem solving (SOLVE)

Treatment Session 5 (end of Week 8)
 Consolidation and rehearsal of skills
 Relapse prevention (targeting techniques for continued application)

Posttreatment assessment

**Outline of Limited-Contact Treatment Over 8 Weeks
(Administration in three clinic sessions)**

Intake assessment

(2–5 weeks of headache self-monitoring)

Treatment Session 1 (beginning of Treatment Week 1)
 Treatment rationale and education about headache
 Progressive muscle relaxation (16 muscle groups)
 Monitoring stressful situations

Scheduled telephone contact (check-in regarding progress, adherence, barriers;
End of Week 1)

Week 2 (no therapist contact)
 Progressive muscle relaxation (7 muscle groups)
 Monitoring stressful situations
 Trigger management

Week 3 (no therapist contact)
 Progressive muscle relaxation (4 muscle groups)
 Monitoring stressful situations
 Trigger management

Week 4 (no therapist contact)
    Progressive muscle relaxation (4 muscle groups, without prerecorded
    instructions)
    Analyzing stressful situations

Treatment Session 2 (beginning of Week 5)
    Thermal biofeedback (optional)
    Relaxation by recall
    Cue-controlled relaxation
    Problem solving (SOLVE)

Week 6 (no therapist contact)
    Thermal biofeedback (optional)
    Relaxation by recall
    Cue-controlled relaxation
    Problem solving (SOLVE)

Scheduled telephone contact (End of Week 6)

Week 7 (no therapist contact)
    Continued relaxation and biofeedback training
    Problem solving (SOLVE)

Treatment Session 3 (end of Week 8)
    Consolidation and rehearsal of skills
    Relapse prevention (targeting techniques for continued application)

Meta-analyses of clinical trials have convincingly demonstrated the utility of these interventions, indicating that for many patients, they are as effective as more intensive behavioral interventions delivered in a specialty clinic (Haddock et al., 1997; Rowan & Andrasik, 1996). A limited-therapist-contact approach, however, may be poorly suited for more complicated patients, including those who are overusing acute headache medications, have significant psychopathology, or have particularly refractory headache presentations.

Limited-contact interventions are more cost-effective over time than even the least expensive prophylactic medications

These limited-contact behavioral therapies are highly cost-competitive when compared with even inexpensive headache medications. To facilitate cost comparisons for pharmacological versus behavioral interventions, in 2011 we reported data on cumulative treatment costs by surveying physicians and behavioral specialists affiliated with the American Headache Society (Schafer et al., 2011). Respondents estimated the costs (e.g., intake, professional fees) of their prototypical regimens for preventive pharmacological treatment, standard clinic-based behavioral treatment, limited-contact behavioral treatment, and group behavioral treatment. Through the first year of treatment, inexpensive prophylactic medications (e.g., beta-blockers or tricyclic antidepressant medications costing less than US $0.75/day) and limited-contact behavioral interventions were the least costly interventions (compared with more costly preventive medications and both standard clinic-based and group behavioral treatments). Thus, relative to pharmacological options, limited-contact behavioral interventions are cost-competitive in the early phases of treatment, and they become the most cost-efficient therapeutic strategy as the years of treatment accrue. (Notably, after 1 year of treatment, even standard clinic-based behavioral treatments are roughly equivalent in cost to preventive medications costing US $1.50/day.) These findings suggest that the expense of behavioral headache interventions is more of a perceived than an actual obstacle to successful implementation in clinical practice.

The newest wave of development for limited-contact therapies includes attempts to integrate highly abbreviated therapies into primary care and use of trained nontherapists to deliver manualized interventions. Preliminary applications of this innovative approach include a single-session intervention with a psychologist, as well as a school-based intervention for pediatric headache by nonpsychologists. Powers and colleagues (2001) reported outcomes from a single session of biofeedback-assisted relaxation training for children as part of a multidisciplinary pediatric headache treatment program. The children were taught age-appropriate relaxation skills and hand warming in a single 1-hr session and given materials for home practice. The patients were able to acquire hand-warming skills in a single session and retain these skills at 15-day follow-up. At follow-up, diary data demonstrated a 25% reduction in headache frequency. Thus, though this was an uncontrolled pilot study, even this single-session behavioral intervention appeared promising.

Likewise, Larsson and colleagues (2005) published data from five studies including 288 children and adolescents over a 20-year period comparing relaxation training taught by either a therapist or school nurse, or using self-help materials as compared with control conditions. Results revealed that the therapist-administered training resulted in the best outcomes, with 60% of children having at least a 50% reduction in headache frequency. Outcomes in groups who received manualized relaxation treatment administered by the school nurse (38% improved) or used self-help materials (30% improved) were superior to control conditions but not as impressive as those in the therapist-administered group. Although these limited studies must be replicated, collectively they demonstrate that limited-contact treatment for headache is a fruitful area of potential dissemination.

4.4.2 Nonprofessionally Administered Treatment

The self-management literature has emphasized use of groups led by trained nonprofessionals who suffer from a chronic disorder. Certification programs have been established for lay leaders, and detailed guides for conducting lay-led but professionally supervised self-management groups for chronic disorders such as arthritis, asthma, diabetes, and chronic back pain have been produced (e.g., http://patienteducation.stanford.edu). Preliminary studies have demonstrated that lay-led migraine self-management groups have potential for yielding at least modest benefit in terms of improved headache outcomes, reduced health care utilization, and enhanced patient SE (Mérelle, Sorbi, van Doornen, & Passchier, 2008; Rothrock et al., 2006).

4.4.3 Self-Help Treatment

Behavioral headache treatments could be made more widely available if patients were able to implement self-management techniques without any face-to-face professional assistance. Few studies to date have evaluated strictly self-help programs, and published studies typically suffer from high attrition rates. For example, one trial reported an impressive 62% reduction in headache at posttreatment (vs. only 14% for "information control"), but the dropout rate exceeded 60% (Kohlenberg & Kahn, 1981). A substantive shortcoming of self-help interventions is the lack of corrective feedback and motivational assistance that patients often need during the initial weeks of skill development and application in their daily routines. Self-help treatments nevertheless may prove beneficial for highly motivated patients with relatively uncomplicated headache problems.

4.4.4   Internet and Mass Communications Treatment

A number of trials have examined headache treatments specifically designed to utilize the Internet and other forms of mass communication. Treatment delivery through such modalities ultimately may allow large numbers of patients to access cost-effective behavioral headache interventions and help overcome the limitations of strictly self-help approaches (Cuijpers, van Straten, & Andersson, 2008). Initial evidence suggests these interventions hold considerable promise for adults (e.g., 40% of migraineurs reported $\geq 50\%$ headache reduction at posttreatment; Hedborg & Muhr, 2011) as well as for children and adolescents (e.g., 63% reported $\geq 50\%$ headache reduction at posttreatment; Trautmann & Kröner-Herwig, 2010). Should a sufficiently large number of patients attain even a modest level of benefit from these interventions, from a public health perspective this approach could have a substantial impact on headache.

4.4.5   Behavioral Interventions Within Medical Practice

Behavioral headache interventions are not well-integrated into routine medical practice

Although the substantial majority of migraineurs who seek care are treated by physicians, self-management principles typically are not well-integrated into routine medical practice. The integration of behavioral self-management principles into physicians' practice settings (both specialty and primary care) is thus a laudable goal that has yet to be fully realized (Penzien et al., 2004). A number of obstacles must be overcome for this integration to take place, including (a) development and validation of referral and treatment algorithms, (b) adaptation of behavioral self-management techniques for these practice settings, (c) development of efficient protocols that allow physicians to integrate self-management training into time-limited patient encounters, and (d) establishing mechanisms for identifying and training the principal coordinators who can deliver these interventions (who may or may not be the physician). Innovative integration of behavioral therapies into physicians' practice settings could be of substantial benefit to headache sufferers who otherwise might not have access to behavioral approaches.

4.5   Problems in Carrying out the Treatments

Tables 18–21 give an overview of common difficulties encountered with relaxation, thermal biofeedback, stress management, and trigger management. Most commonly, problems with the various components of behavioral interventions are a function of patient attitudes or beliefs, difficulty learning the requisite skill, and trouble generalizing gains to everyday experience. The tables also present several simple strategies useful for addressing each problem area (see Tables 18, 19, 20, and 21).

Most difficulties with behavioral treatments can be easily addressed using simple strategies

4.5.1   Difficulties With Relaxation

Table 18
Relaxation Training: Problems and Solutions

Problem area	Strategies for addressing problems
Patient attitudes and beliefs	
Patient makes negative self-statements	• Identify them and help patient to modify them
Patient is overly concerned about her performance in relaxation training exercise	• Suggest patient may be trying too hard and suggest an attitude of passive volition
Patient is hesitant to relinquish control and vigilance	• Discuss concerns about decreasing vigilance and control • Help patient reframe relaxation as a way to gain control, not lose control
Skill development	
Patient is sleepy when practicing relaxation	• Do not schedule relaxation practice just after meals or just before bed-time • Instruct patient to sit upright in a chair during practice
Concentration is disturbed by interfering thoughts and feelings	• Develop imagery techniques (e.g., placing interrupting thoughts in an imaginary closet)
Patient's mind "wanders" during relaxation practice	• Help patient focus attention by repetition of autogenic phrases (e.g., peaceful, calm)
Maintenance and generalization	
Patient reports no carryover effect after relaxation training	• Help patient internalize exercise and develop self-control • Introduce brief cue-controlled techniques that can be used periodically during the day
Patient has difficulty detecting differences between tension and relaxation	• Help patient identify subjective cues of relaxation and tension • Employ relaxation and tension discrimination training

Adapted from Holroyd & Penzien (1993).

4.5.2   Difficulties With Biofeedback

Table 19
Biofeedback Training: Problems and Solutions

Problem area	Strategies for addressing problems
Patient attitudes and beliefs	
Patient does not think she is changing the biofeedback signal	• Encourage patient to adopt an experimenter's attitude • Encourage patient to look at thermometer less often
Patient perceives the task as an achievement challenge	• Assist patient to reappraise the situation and to adopt a more passive approach
Patient is anxious regarding her performance	• Reassure patient about her ability to learn the skill, and allow her to practice without the therapist present to minimize performance anxiety
Skill development	
No change in the thermal response	• Problem-solve with patient to develop a more effective strategy (e.g., add imagery, autogenic phrases) • If using an electronic unit, alter signal threshold to make task easier or use response-shaping techniques to initiate change
Hand temperature decreases rather than increases	• Suggest patient may be trying too hard and encourage a more passive approach • Consider practicing for shorter periods (< 15 min) • Ensure ambient temperature is sufficiently warm
Lack of variability in the patient's hand temperature makes biofeedback difficult	• Investigate potential physiological effects of patient's medications (e.g., propranolol) • Advise patient it can be challenging to raise hand temperature above 90 °F (32 °C).
Maintenance and generalization	
Patient shows considerable variability in control from one clinic training session to the next	• Emphasize home practice to help reduce between-session variability
Patient has difficulty recognizing subjective cues and is dependent on feedback signal for indication of success	• Help patient identify subjective cues of success • Emphasize importance of developing self-control skills

Adapted from Holroyd & Penzien (1993).

4.5.3 Difficulties With Stress Management

Table 20
Stress Management Training: Problems and Solutions

Problem area	Techniques for addressing problems
Patient attitudes and beliefs	
Patient fails to recognize that her behavior can influence stress responses or headache activity	• Review the rationale for stress management • Solicit real-world examples to illustrate how behaviors and cognitions can influence stress responses
Patient lacks confidence in her ability to self-manage her headaches	• Address faulty beliefs that headaches are outside her control or reflect a personal deficiency • Attend to patient's actual as well as perceived performance during skills training • Provide positive reinforcement by accentuating the value of even small successes
Skill development	
Patient reveals a large number of different stressful situations	• Isolate common themes that cut across multiple problems • List problems from least to worst and begin working on a manageable problem first • Encourage maintenance of focus on selected problem
Headaches are not obviously stress-related or patient has difficulty identifying stressors	• Review headache self-monitoring and analyze situations associated with headache • Reference physical cues, events, or times associated with headache and probe to identify concrete behaviors and thoughts • Consider using events in therapy to help identify stressors • Emphasize biofeedback more than stress management
Headache is always present so headache triggers can prove difficult to identify	• Identify factors associated with exacerbation rather than onset of headache
Patient's and therapist's preferred target problems differ	• Openly discuss difference of opinion • Defer to patient if patient has strong preference

Table 20 (continued)

Problem area	Techniques for addressing problems
Friction is present in therapeutic relationship	• Openly discuss conflict • Examine conflict as cues to patient's coping style • Assume responsibility for therapist errors
Maintenance and generalization	
Patient does not attempt or attempts but "fails" homework assignment	• Reiterate importance of regular practice • Examine maladaptive beliefs about homework • Frame assignments as an opportunity to learn • Assist with time management and prioritization • Break assignments into smaller, more manageable tasks
Patient attributes lack of change to external factors (e.g., inflexibility in employment)	• Identify cognitions that prevent patient from seeing alternatives • Encourage experimentation with "small changes" • Assist the patient to identify "adaptive copers" among acquaintances as models of feasible change
Patient believes maladaptive thoughts to be self-evidently true	• Offer a variety of alternative explanations of the same "facts" • Reverse roles to encourage taking alternative perspective

Adapted from Holroyd, K. A., Lipchik, G. L., & Penzien, D. B. (1998). Psychological management of recurrent headache disorders: Empirical basis for clinical practice. In K. S. Dobson & K. D. Craig (Eds.), *Best practice: Developing and promoting empirically supported interventions* (pp. 187–235). Newbury Park, CA: Sage. © SAGE. Reprinted with permission.

4.5.4   Difficulties With Trigger Management

Table 21
Trigger Management Training: Problems and Solutions

Problem area	Strategies for addressing problems
Patient attitudes and beliefs	
Patient is overwhelmed by large number of possible trigger factors	• Focus first on most common triggers among headache patients • Prioritize 2–3 personal triggers that are most salient • Extend duration of trigger self-monitoring to identify themes over longer time periods
Patient lacks confidence to manage triggers	• Remind patient even modest lifestyle adjustments to reduce exposure to relevant triggers can prove beneficial • Help patient identify triggers most amenable to modification • Prioritize 2–3 personal triggers that are most common or salient
Skill development	
Patient cannot identify whether a potential trigger is personally relevant	• Encourage patient to adopt an "experimenter's attitude" as she examines trigger factors • Use behavioral experiments • Remind patient there may be a delay or "lag" between trigger exposure and headache onset
Headache is always present so headache triggers can prove difficult to identify	• Identify trigger factors potentially associated with exacerbation rather than onset of headache
Maintenance and generalization	
Patient is unable to manage certain trigger(s) in everyday life	• Assess frequency of skills practice outside the clinic • Consider whether the trigger is interacting with another trigger that has been overlooked • Help the patient realize that some triggers are uncontrollable (e.g., weather) and help her work to predict and prepare for these triggers or implement acceptance-based strategies

4.6   Multicultural Issues

As discussed in Section 1.3, migraine is predominantly a women's health issue, affecting women three times more often than men. Although both migraine and TTH are slightly less common among racial and ethnic minority groups than among Whites, prevalence of migraine is highest among those of lower SES. However, racial and ethnic disparities in health care quality and access are well documented, and these disparities likely occur in part because of associations between race/ethnicity and SES. As such, racial and ethnic minorities are perhaps less likely to receive an appropriate migraine diagnosis and subsequent treatment. Although Black Americans often report more frequent and severe headaches than White Americans (Heckman, Merrill, & Anderson, 2013) and are more likely to terminate headache treatment prematurely (Heckman et al., 2008; 2009), individuals of both races respond equally well when treated within headache specialty centers. These findings suggest that ensuring better access to quality headache treatments, whether pharmacological or behavioral, can greatly facilitate positive outcomes among minority headache patients.

5

Conclusion

Migraine and TTH are common and disabling conditions that are influenced by a host of behavioral and psychological variables. Despite widespread availability of efficacious preventive and acute pharmacotherapies for migraine, many headache patients prefer behavioral interventions to medication, and for other patients, pharmacotherapy is contraindicated. Supplementing pharmacotherapy with behavioral interventions also produces outcomes superior to those for either treatment alone. The efficacy of behavioral headache interventions for both migraine and TTH has been firmly established over the past 4 decades, both in numerous clinical trials and in multiple meta-analyses of these trials.

Behavioral headache therapies are informed by a biopsychosocial perspective of headache, in which headache is conceptualized as a neurological disorder, the triggering and maintenance of which is strongly influenced by behavioral and lifestyle factors. Behavioral interventions principally target stress and physiological changes that commonly precede headache onset. The underlying theme is that patients can learn to actively self-manage their headache problem to reduce the likelihood of future attacks and minimize associated disability.

The major components of behavioral headache therapies are relaxation training, biofeedback training, and stress management training. Relaxation and biofeedback aim to reduce physiological arousal that can accompany primary headache disorders, and stress management training is designed to reduce stress and improve coping skills. Health behavior education and self-monitoring are integrated into each of these three major intervention components. Many patients benefit also from behavioral approaches that emphasize formal management of specific headache triggers, facilitating adherence to pharmacotherapy and behavioral change, and acceptance-based strategies. Each of these interventions has been detailed in this volume, with accompanying forms and handouts in the Appendix.

By considering unique patient and contextual factors reviewed in this volume, the mental health provider can develop and implement an empirically based behavioral treatment that is individually tailored for each headache patient.

6

Further Reading

Lake, A. E., III, Lipchik, G. L., Penzien, D. B., Rains, J. C., Saper, J. R., & Lipton, R. B. (Eds.). (2006). Psychiatric comorbidity with chronic headache: Evidence-based clinical implications [Supplement]. *Headache, 46,* S73–S167.

Penzien, D. B., Rains, J. C., Lake, A. E., Lipchik, G. L., Lipton, R. B., & Saper, J. R. (Eds.). (2006). Complex comorbidities of recurrent headache disorders [Special Series]. *Headache, 46*(9), 1323–1423. doi: 10.1111/j.1526-4610.2006.00575.x

The psychiatric comorbidity Special Series and Supplement were published in tandem to improve the care of headache patients who have a comorbid psychiatric disorder. The collection of comprehensive literature reviews in the Special Series summarizes epidemiological and clinical research pertaining to psychiatric disorders among patients with recurrent headache disorders. The Supplement contains more applied articles that integrate the scientific literature with empirically based recommendations pertaining to assessment and treatment of these complex patients.

Olesen, J., Goadsby, P. J., Ramadan, N. M., Tfelt-Hansen, P., & Welch, K. M. A. (2006). *The Headaches* (3rd ed.). Philadelphia, PA: Lippincott, Williams, & Wilkins.

This book is an encyclopedic reference with contributions by many of the foremost international authorities on headache; it provides evidence-based treatment recommendations and includes extensive tables of relevant controlled clinical trials.

Penzien, D. B. (Ed.). (2005). Guidelines for trials of behavioral treatments for recurrent headache [Supplement]. *Headache, 45*(5), S87–S132 doi: 10.1111/j.1526-4610.2005.4502001.x

Penzien, D. B., & Maizels, M. (Eds.). (2005). Headache research methodology [Special Series]. *Headache, 45*(5), 408–537. doi: 10.1111/j.1526-4610.2005.05090.x

The behavioral clinical trials guidelines presented in this Supplement and Special Series were developed to enhance the quality and consistency of research evaluating behavioral treatments for primary headache disorders. Developed under the auspices of the American Headache Society (AHS), the guidelines are complementary to, and modeled after, guidelines published by the International Headache Society to address research methodology appropriate for drug trials for headache. The guidelines are complemented by a Special Series of articles addressing headache research methodology, with each individual article focusing on a key research design and methodological issue confronting headache investigators. The Series also presents an authoritative review of the behavioral headache treatment literature accompanied by a critique of the methodological quality of that literature, as well as a paper enumerating unmet needs and priorities for evaluating behavioral headache therapies.

Schulman, E. A., Levin, M., Lake, A. E., III, & Loder, E. (Eds.). (2010). *Refractory migraine: Mechanisms and management.* New York, NY: Oxford University Press.

International experts from top headache centers describe how they approach management of migraine patients who continue to suffer despite appropriate medical care. The text presents current concepts regarding the characterization of "refractory migraine," including underlying causes and contributing factors, and then gives an overview of treatment strategies focused specifically upon refractory forms of the disorder. The volume includes detailed algorithms for outpatient and inpatient withdrawal from overused medications, innovative drug therapies and nonpharmacological treatments, considerations before implementing hormonal therapies, and how to approach patients with personality disorders or other psychiatric comorbidities.

Silberstein, S. D., Lipton, R. B., & Dodick, D. W. (Eds.). (2008). *Wolff's headache and other head pain* (8th ed.). New York, NY: Oxford University Press.
For decades this book has served as the definitive reference for "everything headache," beginning with Wolff's first edition in 1948. The current volume includes 34 chapters focusing on diagnosis and treatment of both primary and secondary headache disorders, as well as special topics such as headache in special populations, behavioral management, and communication with patients.

7

References

American Psychiatric Association. (2013). *Diagnostic and statistical manual of mental disorders* (*5th ed.*). Washington, DC: Author.

Andrasik, F., & Holroyd, K. A. (1980). A test of specific and nonspecific effects in the biofeedback treatment of tension headache. *Journal of Consulting and Clinical Psychology, 48,* 575–586. doi: 10.1037/0022-006X.48.5.575

Andrasik, F., & Holroyd, K. A. (1983). Specific and nonspecific effects in the biofeedback treatment of tension headache: 3-year follow-up. *Journal of Consulting and Clinical Psychology, 51,* 634–636. doi: 10.1037/0022-006X.51.4.634

Andrew, M. E., Penzien, D. B., Rains, J. C., Knowlton, G. E., & McAnulty, R. D. (1992). Development of a computer application for headache diagnosis: The Headache Diagnostic System. *International Journal of Biomedical Computing, 31,* 17–24. doi: 10.1016/0020-7101(92)90050-3

Ashkenazi, V., Levin, M., & Dodick, D. W. (2008). Peripheral procedures: Nerve blocks, peripheral neurostimulation, and botulinum neurotoxin injections. In S. D. Silberstein, R. B. Lipton, & D. W. Dodick (Eds.), *Wolff's headache and other head pain* (8th ed., pp. 767–792). New York, NY: Oxford University Press.

Bandura, A. (1997). *Self-efficacy: The exercise of control.* New York, NY: W.H. Freeman.

Bandura, A., Cioffi, D., Taylor, C. B., & Brouillard, M. E. (1988). Perceived self-efficacy in coping with cognitive stressors and opioid activation. *Journal of Personality and Social Psychology, 55,* 479–488. doi: 10.1037/0022-3514.55.3.479

Baskin, S. M., & Smitherman, T. A. (2009). Migraine and psychiatric disorders: comorbidities, mechanisms, and clinical applications. *Neurological Sciences, 30*(Suppl 1), 61–65. doi: 10.1007/s10072-009-0071-5

Bernstein, D. A., & Borkovec, T. D. (1973). *Progressive relaxation training: A manual for the helping professions.* Champaign, IL: Research Press.

Bigal, M. E., Liberman, J. N., & Lipton, R. B. (2006). Obesity and migraine: A population study. *Neurology, 66,* 545–550. doi: 10.1212/01.wnl.0000197218.05284.82

Bigal, M. E., Kurth, T., Santanello, N., Buse, D., Golden, W., Robbins, & Lipton, R. B. (2010). Migraine and cardiovascular disease: A population-based study. *Neurology, 74,* 628–635. doi: 10.1212/WNL.0b013e3181d0cc8b

Blanchard, E. B. (1992). Psychological treatment of benign headache disorders. *Journal of Consulting and Clinical Psychology, 60,* 537–551. doi: 10.1037/0022-006X.60.4.537

Blanchard, E. B., Andrasik, F., Evans, D. D., & Hillhouse, J. (1985). Biofeedback and relaxation treatments for headache in the elderly: A caution and a challenge. *Applied Psychophysiology and Biofeedback, 10,* 69–73.

Blanchard, E. B., Appelbaum, K. A., Guarnieri, P., Morrill, B., & Dentinger, M.P. (1987). Five year prospective follow-up on the treatment of chronic headache with biofeedback and/or relaxation. *Headache, 27,* 580–583. doi: 10.1111/j.1526-4610.1987.hed2710580.x

Borckardt, J. J., Nash, M. R., Murphy, M. D., Moore, M., Shaw, D., & O'Neil, P. (2008). Clinical practice as natural laboratory for psychotherapy research: a guide to case-based time-series analysis. *American Psychologist, 63,* 77–95. doi: 10.1037/0003-066X.63.2.77

Breslau, N. (1998). Psychiatric comorbidity in migraine. *Cephalalgia, 18*(Suppl 22), S56–S61.

Breslau, N., Lipton, R. B., Stewart, W. F., Schultz, L. R., & Welch, K. M. A. (2003). Comorbidity of migraine and major depression: Investigating potential etiology and prognosis. *Neurology, 60,* 1308–1312. doi: 10.1212/01.WNL.0000058907.41080.54

Breslau, N., Schultz, L., Lipton, R., Peterson, E., & Welch, K. M. A. (2012). Migraine headaches and suicide attempt. *Headache, 52*, 723–731. doi: 10.1111/j.1526-4610.2012.02117.x

Brønfort, G., Nilsson, N., Haas, M., Evans, R. L., Goldsmith, C. H., Assendelft, W. J. J., & Bouter, L. M. (2009). Non-invasive physical treatments for chronic/recurrent headache. *Cochrane Database of Systematic Reviews, 3,* CD001878. doi: 10.1002/14651858. CD001878.pub2

Budzynski, T. H., & Stoyva, J. M. (1969). An instrument for producing deep muscle relaxation by means of analog information feedback. *Journal of Applied Behavioral Analysis, 2,* 231–237. doi: 10.1901/jaba.1969.2-231

Calhoun, A. H., & Ford, S. (2007). Behavioral sleep modification may revert transformed migraine to episodic migraine. *Headache, 47,* 1178–1183. doi: 10.1111/j.1526-4610.2007.00780.x

Campbell, J. K., Penzien, D. B., & Wall, E. M. (2000). *Evidence-based guidelines for migraine headache: Behavioral and physical treatments* [Online]. Retrieved from http://www.americanheadachesociety.org/assets/1/7/04_HAConsortium_BehavioralGuideline2000.PDF

Cram, J. R. (1980). EMG biofeedback and the treatment of tension headaches: A systematic analysis of treatment components. *Headache, 11,* 699–710.

Cuijpers, P., van Straten, A., & Andersson, G. (2008). Internet-administered cognitive behavior therapy for health problems: A systematic review. *Journal of Behavioral Medicine, 31,* 169–177. doi: 10.1007/s10865-007-9144-1

Davis, M. K., Holroyd, K. A., & Penzien, D. B. (1999). Flunarizine and propranolol: Comparative effectiveness in the treatment of migraine headaches. *Headache, 39,* 349.

Detsky, M. E., McDonald, D. R., Baerlocher, M. O., Tomlinson, G. A., McCrory, D. C., & Booth, C. M. (2006). Does this patient with headache have a migraine or need neuroimaging? *JAMA, 296,* 1274–1283. doi: 10.1001/jama.296.10.1274

Dindo, L., Recober, A., Marchman, J., O'Hara, M. W., & Turvey, C. (2014). One-day behavioral intervention in depressed migraine patients: Effects on headache. *Headache, 54,* 528–538. doi: 10.1111/head.12258

Dindo, L., Recober, A., Marchman, J. N., Turvey, C., & O'Hara, M. W. (2012). One-day behavioral treatment for patients with comorbid depression and migraine: A pilot study. *Behaviour Research and Therapy, 50,* 537–543. doi: 10.1016/j.brat.2012.05.007

Dodick, D. W. (2003). Diagnosing headache: Clinical cues and clinical rules. *Advanced Studies in Medicine, 3,* 87–92.

Dodick, D. W. (2009). Review of comorbidities and risk factors for the development of migraine complications (infarct and chronic migraine). *Cephalalgia, 29*(Suppl 3), 7–14. doi: 10.1177/03331024090290S303

Engel, G. L. (1977). The need for a new medical model: A challenge for biomedicine. *Science, 196,* 129–136. doi: 10.1126/science.847460

Ford, S., Calhoun, A., Kahn, K., Mann, J., Finkel, A. (2008). Predictors of disability in migraineurs referred to a tertiary clinic: neck pain, headache characteristics, and coping behaviors. *Headache, 48,* 523–528. doi: 10.1111/j.1526-4610.2008.00859.x

French, D. J., Holroyd, K. A., Pinell, C., Malinoski, P. T., O'Donnell, F., & Hill, K. R. (2000). Perceived self-efficacy and headache-related disability. *Headache, 40,* 647–656. doi: 10.1046/j.1526-4610.2000.040008647.x

Goadsby, P. J., Charbit, A. R., Andreou, A. P., Akerman, S., & Holland, P. R. (2009). Neurobiology of migraine. *Neuroscience, 161,* 327–341. doi: 10.1016/j.neuroscience.2009.03.019

Goadsby, P. J., Lipton, R. B., & Ferrari, M. D. (2002). Migraine: Current understanding and treatment. *New England Journal of Medicine, 346,* 257–270. doi: 10.1056/NEJMra010917

Goslin, R. E., Gray, R. N., McCrory, D. C., Penzien, D., Rains, J., Hasselblad, V. (1999). Behavioral and physical treatments for migraine headache. In Agency for Healthcare Research and Quality, *Technical Reviews 2.2.* Rockville, MD: Agency for Health Care Policy and Research. Retrieved from http://www.ncbi.nlm.nih.gov/books/NBK45267/?part

Haddock, C. K., Rowan, A. B., Andrasik, F., Wilson, P. G., Talcott, G. W., & Stein, R. J. (1997). Home-based behavioral treatments for chronic benign headache: A meta-analysis of controlled trials. *Cephalalgia, 17,* 113–118. doi: 10.1046/j.1468-2982.1997.1702113.x

Hamel, E. (2007). Serotonin and migraine: Biology and clinical implications. *Cephalalgia, 27*, 1295–1300. doi: 10.1111/j.1468-2982.2007.01476.x

Hamelsky, S. W., & Lipton, R. B. (2006). Psychiatric comorbidity of migraine. *Headache, 46*, 1327–1333. doi: 10.1111/j.1526-4610.2006.00576.x

Hassinger, H. J., Semenchuk, E. M., & O'Brien, W. H. (1999). Appraisal and coping responses to pain and stress in migraine headache sufferers. *Journal of Behavioral Medicine, 22*, 327– 340. doi: 10.1023/A:1018722002393

Headache Classification Committee of the International Headache Society. (2013). The International Classification of Headache Disorders (3rd ed., beta version). *Cephalalgia, 33*, 629–808. doi: 10.1177/0333102413485658

Heckman, B. D., & Holroyd, K. A. (2006). Tension-type headache and psychiatric comorbidity. *Current Pain and Headache Reports, 10*, 439–447. doi: 10.1007/s11916-006-0075-2

Heckman, B. D., Holroyd, K. A., O'Donnell, F. J., Tietjen, G., Utley, C., Stillman, M., ... Ellis, G. (2008). Race differences in adherence to headache treatment appointments in persons with headache disorders. *Journal of the National Medical Association, 100*, 247–255.

Heckman, B. D., Holroyd, K. A., Tietjen, G., O'Donnell, F. J., Himawan, L., Utley, C., ... Stillman, M. (2009). Whites and African-Americans in headache specialty clinics respond equally well to treatment. *Cephalalgia, 29*, 650–661. doi: 10.1111/j.1468-2982.2008.01785.x

Heckman, B. D., Merrill, J. C., & Anderson, T. (2013). Race, psychiatric comorbidity, and headache characteristics in patients in headache subspecialty treatment clinics. *Ethnicity and Health, 18*, 34–52. doi: 10.1080/13557858.2012.682219

Hedborg, K., & Muhr, C. (2011). Multimodal behavioral treatment of migraine: an Internet-administered, randomized, controlled trial. *Upsala Journal of Medical Sciences, 116*, 169–186. doi: 10.3109/03009734.2011.575963

Holland, S., Silberstein, S. D., Freitag, F., Dodick, D. W., Argoff, C., & Ashman, E. (2012). Evidence-based guideline update: NSAIDs and other complementary treatments for episodic migraine prevention in adults: Report of the Quality Standards Subcommittee of the American Academy of Neurology and the American Headache Society. *Neurology, 78*, 1346–1353. doi: 10.1212/WNL.0b013e3182535d0c

Holm, J. E., Holroyd, K. A., Hursey, K. G., & Penzien, D. B. (1986). The role of stress in recurrent tension headache. *Headache, 26*, 160–167. doi: 10.1111/j.1526-4610.1986.hed2604160.x

Holm, J. E., Penzien, D. B., Holroyd, K. A., & Brown, T. A. (1994). Headache and depression: Confounding effects of transdiagnostic symptoms. *Headache, 34*, 418–422. doi: 10.1111/j.1526-4610.1994.hed3407418.x

Holroyd, K. A. (2002). Assessment and psychological management of recurrent headache disorders. *Journal of Consulting and Clinical Psychology, 70*, 656–677. doi: 10.1037/0022-006X.70.3.656

Holroyd, K. A., Cottrell, C. K., O'Donnell, F. J., Cordingley, G. E., Drew, J. B., Carlson, B. W., & Himawan, L. (2010). Effect of preventive (beta blocker) treatment, behavioural migraine management, or their combination on outcomes of optimised acute treatment in frequent migraine: randomised controlled trial. *British Medical Journal, 341*, c4871. doi: 10.1136/bmj.c4871

Holroyd, K. A., Lipchik, G. L., & Penzien, D. B. (1998). Psychological management of recurrent headache disorders: Empirical basis for clinical practice. In K. S. Dobson & K. D. Craig (Eds.), *Best practice: Developing and promoting empirically supported interventions* (pp. 187–235). Newbury Park, CA: Sage.

Holroyd, K. A., O'Donnell, F. J., Stensland, M., Lipchik, G. L., Cordingley, G. E., & Carlson, B. W. (2001). Management of chronic tension-type headache with tricyclic antidepressant medication, stress management therapy, and their combination: A randomized controlled trial. *Journal of the American Medical Association, 285*, 2208–2215. doi: 10.1001/jama.285.17.2208

Holroyd, K. A., & Penzien, D. B. (1986). Client variables and the behavioral treatment of recurrent tension headache: A meta-analytic review. *Journal of Behavioral Medicine, 9,* 515–536. doi: 10.1007/BF00845282

Holroyd, K. A., & Penzien, D. B. (1990). Pharmacological vs. nonpharmacological prophylaxis of recurrent migraine headache: A meta-analytic review of clinical trials. *Pain, 42,* 1–13. doi: 10.1016/0304-3959(90)91085-W

Holroyd, K. A., & Penzien, D. B. (1993). *Self-management of recurrent headache.* Geneva, Switzerland: World Health Organization.

Holroyd, K. A., Penzien, D. B., Hursey, K. G., Tobin, D. L., Roger, L., Holm, J. E., … Chila, A. G. (1984). Change mechanisms in EMG biofeedback training: Cognitive changes underlying improvement in tension headache. *Journal of Consulting and Clinical Psychology, 52,* 1039–1054. doi: 10.1037/0022-006X.52.6.1039

Houle, T. T., Butschek, R. A., Turner, D. P., Smitherman, T. A., Rains, J. C., & Penzien, D. P. (2012). Stress and sleep predict headache severity in chronic headache sufferers. *Pain, 153,* 2432–2440. doi: 10.1016/j.pain.2012.08.014

Houle, T. T., & Nash, J. M. (2008). Stress and headache chronification. *Headache, 48,* 40–44. doi: 10.1111/j.1526-4610.2007.00973.x

Houle, T. T., Remble, T. A., & Houle, T. A. (2005). The examination of headache activity using time-series research designs. *Headache, 45,* 438–444. doi: 10.1111/j.1526-4610.2005.05095.x

Houle, T. T., Turner, D. P., Smitherman, T. A., Penzien, D. B., & Lipton, R. B. (2013). Influence of random measurement error on estimated rates of headache chronification and remission. *Headache, 53,* 920–929. doi: 10.1111/head.12125

Hudzynski, L., & Levenson, H. (1985). Biofeedback behavioral treatment of headache with locus of control pain analysis: A 20-month retrospective study. *Headache, 25,* 380–386. doi: 10.1111/j.1526-4610.1985.hed2507380.x

Jacobson, E. (1938). *Progressive relaxation.* Chicago, IL: University of Chicago Press.

Jacobson, G. P., Ramadan, N. M., Aggarwal, S. K., & Newman, C. W. (1994). The Henry Ford Hospital Headache Disability Inventory (HDI). *Neurology, 44,* 837–842. doi: 10.1212/WNL.44.5.837

Jackson, J. L., Kuriyama, A., & Hayashino, Y. (2012). Botulinum toxin A for prophylactic treatment of migraine and tension headaches in adults. *JAMA, 307,* 1736–1745. doi: 10.1001/jama.2012.505

Jhingran, P., Osterhouse, J. T., Miller, D. W., Lee, J. T., & Kirchdoerfer, L. (1998). Development and validation of the migraine-specific quality of life questionnaire. *Headache, 38,* 295–302. doi: 10.1046/j.1526-4610.1998.3804295.x

Juang, K. D., Wang, S. J., Fuh, J. L., Lu, S. R., & Su, T. P. (2000). Comorbidity of depressive and anxiety disorders in chronic daily headache and its subtypes. *Headache, 40,* 818–823. doi: 10.1046/j.1526-4610.2000.00148.x

Keefe, F. J., Affleck, G., Lefebvre, J. C., Starr, K., Caldwell, D. S., & Tennen, H. (1997). Pain coping strategies and coping efficacy in rheumatoid arthritis: A daily process analysis. *Pain, 69,* 35–42. doi: 10.1016/S0304-3959(96)03246-0

Keefe, F. J., Rumble, M. E., Scipio, C. D., Giordano, L. A., & Perri, L. M. (2004). Psychological aspects of persistent pain: Current state of the science. *Journal of Pain, 5,* 195–211. doi: 10.1016/j.jpain.2004.02.576

Kelman, L. (2007). The triggers or precipitants of the acute migraine attack. *Cephalalgia, 27,* 394–402. doi: 10.1111/j.1468-2982.2007.01303.x

Kelman, L., & Rains, J. C. (2005). Headache and sleep: Examination of sleep patterns and complaints in a large clinical sample of migraineurs. *Headache, 45,* 904–910. doi: 10.1111/j.1526-4610.2005.05159.x

Kohlenberg, R. J., & Kahn, T. (1981). Self-help treatment for migraine headaches: A controlled outcome study. *Headache, 21,* 196–200. doi: 10.1111/j.1526-4610.1981.hed2105196.x

Kosinski, M., Bayliss, M. S., Bjorner, J. B., Ware Jr, J. E., Garber, W. H., Baterhorst, A., … Tepper, S. (2003). A six-item short-form survey for measuring headache impact: The HIT-6. *Quality of Life Research, 12,* 963–974. doi: 10.1023/A:1026119331193

Kroenke, K., Spitzer, R. L., & Williams, J. B. (2001). The PHQ-9: Validity of a brief depression screening measure. *Journal of General Internal Medicine, 16*, 606–613. doi: 10.1046/j.1525-1497.2001.016009606.x

Kroenke, K., Spitzer, R. L., Williams, J. B. W., Monahan, P. O., & Löwe, B. (2007). Anxiety disorders in primary care: Prevalence, impairment, comorbidity, and detection. *Annals of Internal Medicine, 146*, 317–325. doi: 10.7326/0003-4819-146-5-200703060-00004

Lake, A. E., III, Saper, J. R., & Hamel, R. L. (2009). Comprehensive inpatient treatment of refractory chronic daily headache. *Headache, 49*, 555–562. doi: 10.1111/j.1526-4610.2009.01364.x

Larsson, B., Carlsson, J., Fichtel, A., & Melin, L. (2005). Relaxation treatment of adolescent headache sufferers: results from a school-based replication series. *Headache, 45*, 692–704. doi: 10.1111/j.1526-4610.2005.05138.x

Lazarus, R. S., & Folkman, S. (1984). *Stress, appraisal, and coping*. New York, NY: Springer.

Linde, K., Allais, G., Brinkhaus, B., Manheimer, E., Vickers, A., & White, A. R. (2009a). Acupuncture for migraine prophylaxis. *Cochrane Database of Systematic Reviews, 1*, CD001218. doi: 10.1002/14651858.CD001218.pub2

Linde, K., Allais, G., Brinkhaus, B., Manheimer, E., Vickers, A., & White, A. R. (2009b). Acupuncture for tension-type headache. *Cochrane Database of Systematic Reviews, 1*, CD007587. doi: 10.1002/14651858.CD007587

Lipchik, G. L., Smitherman, T. A., Penzien, D. B., & Holroyd, K. (2006). Basic principles and techniques of cognitive-behavioral therapies for comorbid psychiatric symptoms among headache patients. *Headache, 46*(Suppl 3), 119–132. doi: 10.1111/j.1526-4610.2006.00563.x

Lipton, R. B., Bigal, M. E., Diamond, M., Freitag, F., Reed, M. L., & Stewart, W. F. (2007). Migraine prevalence, disease burden, and the need for preventive therapy. *Neurology, 68*, 343–349. doi: 10.1212/01.wnl.0000252808.97649.21

Lipton, R. B., Bigal, M. E., Hamelsky, S., & Scher, A. I. (2008). Headache: Epidemiology and impact. In S. Silberstein, R. Lipton, & D. Dodick (Eds.), *Wolff's headache and other head pain (8th ed.*, pp. 45–62). New York, NY: Oxford University Press.

Lipton, R. B., Silberstein, S. D., Saper, J. R., Bigal, M. E., & Goadsby, P. J. (2003). Why headache treatment fails. *Neurology, 60*, 1064–1070. doi: 10.1212/01.WNL.0000052687.03646.74

Lipton, R. B., Stewart, W. F., & Simon, D. (1998). Medical consultation for migraine: Results from the American Migraine Study. *Headache, 38*, 87–96. doi: 10.1046/j.1526-4610.1998.3802087.x

Maizels, M., Aurora, S., & Heinricher, M. (2012). Beyond neurovascular: Migraine as a dysfunctional neurolimbic pain network. *Headache, 10*, 1553–1565. doi: 10.1111/j.1526-4610.2012.02209.x

Maizels, M., Smitherman, T. A., & Penzien, D. B. (2006). A review of screening tools for psychiatric comorbidity in headache patients. *Headache, 46*(Suppl 3), 98–109. doi: 10.1111/j.1526-4610.2006.00561.x

Martin, N. J., Holroyd, K. A., & Penzien, D. B. (1990). The headache-specific locus of control scale: Adaptation to recurrent headaches. *Headache, 30*, 729–734. doi: 10.1111/j.1526-4610.1990.hed3011729.x

Martin, N. J., Holroyd, K. A., & Rokicki, L. A. (1993). The Headache Self-Efficacy Scale: Adaptation to recurrent headaches. *Headache, 33*, 244–248. doi: 10.1111/j.1526-4610.1993.hed3305244.x

Martin, P. R. (1993). *Psychological management of chronic headaches*. New York, NY: Guilford.

Martin, P. R., & MacLeod, C. (2009). Behavioral management of headache triggers: Avoidance of triggers is an inadequate strategy. *Clinical Psychology Review, 29*, 483–495. doi: 10.1016/j.cpr.2009.05.002

Martin, V. T., & Behbehani, V. T. (2006). Ovarian hormones and migraine headache: Understanding mechanisms and pathogenesis: Part I. *Headache, 46*, 3–23. doi: 10.1111/j.1526-4610.2006.00370.x

Matchar, D. B., Young, W. B., Rosenberg, J. H., Pietrzak, M. P., Silberstein, R. B., & Ramadan, N. M. (2000). *Evidence-based guidelines for migraine headache in the primary care setting: Pharmacological management of acute attacks* [Online]. Retrieved from http://tools.aan.com/professionals/practice/pdfs/gl0087.pdf

McCrory, D. C., Penzien, D. B., Hasselblad, V., & Gray, R.N. (2001). *Evidence report: Behavioral and physical treatments for tension-type and cervicogenic headache.* Product No. 2085. Des Moines, IA: Foundation for Chiropractic Education and Research.

Mérelle, S. Y., Sorbi, M. J., van Doornen, L. J., & Passchier, J. (2008). Lay trainers with migraine for a home-based behavioral training: A 6-month follow-up study. *Headache, 48,* 1311–1325. doi: 10.1111/j.1526-4610.2007.01043.x

Mo'tamedi, H., Rezaiemaram, P., & Tavallaie, A. (2012). The effectiveness of a group-based acceptance and commitment additive therapy on rehabilitation of female outpatients with chronic headache: Preliminary findings reducing 3 dimensions of headache impact. *Headache, 52,* 1106–1119. doi: 10.1111/j.1526-4610.2012.02192.x

Moja, L., Cusi, C., Sterzi, R., & Canepari, C. (2005). Selective serotonin re-uptake inhibitors (SSRIs) for preventing migraine and tension-type headaches. *Cochrane Database of Systematic Reviews, 3,* CD002919. doi: 10.1002/14651858.CD002919.pub2

Mosley, T. H., Grotheus, C. A., & Meeks, W. M. (1995). Treatment of tension headache in the elderly: A controlled evaluation of relaxation training and relaxation combined with cognitive-behavior therapy. *Journal of Clinical Geropsychology, 1,* 175–188.

Nash, J. R., & Thebarge, R. W. (2006). Understanding psychological stress, its biological processes, and impact on primary headache. *Headache, 46,* 1377–1386. doi: 10.1111/j.1526-4610.2006.00580.x

Nestoriuc, Y., & Martin, A. (2007). Efficacy of biofeedback for migraine: A meta-analysis. *Pain, 128,* 111–127. doi: 10.1016/j.pain.2006.09.007

Nestoriuc, Y., Rief, W., & Martin, A. (2008). Meta-analysis of biofeedback for tension-type headache: Efficacy, specificity, and treatment moderators. *Journal of Consulting and Clinical Psychology, 76,* 379–396. doi: 10.1037/0022-006X.76.3.379

Nicholson, R. A., Houle, T. T., Rhudy, J. L., & Norton, P. J. (2007). Psychological risk factors in headache. *Headache, 47,* 413–426.

Nicholson, R. A., Nash, J., & Andrasik, F. A. (2005). A self-administered behavioral intervention using tailored messages for migraine. *Headache, 45,* 1124–1139. doi: 10.1111/j.1526-4610.2005.00236.x

Palermo, T. M., Eccleston, C., Lewandowski, A. S., Williams, A. C., & Morley, S. (2010). Randomized controlled trials of psychological therapies for management of chronic pain in children and adolescents: An updated meta-analytic review. *Pain, 148,* 387–397. doi: 10.1016/j.pain.2009.10.004

Penzien, D. B., Andrasik, F., Freidenberg, B. M., Houle, T. T., Lake, A. E., . . . Wittrock, D. A. (2005). Guidelines for trials of behavioral treatments for recurrent headache. *Headache, 45,* S109–S131. doi: 10.1111/j.1526-4610.2005.4502001.x

Penzien, D. B., Johnson, C. A., Seville, J., Rubman, S., Boggess, J. T., & Rains, J. C. (1994). Interrelationships among daily and global self-report measures of headache. *Headache Quarterly, 5,* 8–14.

Penzien, D. B., & Rains, J. C. (2005). How behavioral headache treatments can help you fine-tune outcomes. *Practical Neurology, 4,* 40–46, 49.

Penzien, D. B., Rains, J. C., & Holroyd, K. A. (1993). Psychological assessment of the recurrent headache sufferer. In C. D. Tollison & R. S. Kunkel (Eds.), *Headache: Diagnosis and treatment* (pp. 39–49). Baltimore, MD: Williams and Wilkins.

Penzien, D. B., Rains, J. C., Lipchik, G. L., & Creer, T. L. (2004). Behavioral interventions for tension-type headache: Overview of current therapies and recommendation for a self-management model for chronic headache. *Current Pain and Headache Reports, 8,* 489–499. doi: 10.1007/s11916-004-0072-2

Penzien, D. B., Rains, J. C., & Lipton, R. B. (2008). Introduction to the special series on the chronification of headache: mechanisms, risk factors, and behavioral strategies aimed at primary and secondary prevention of chronic headache. *Headache, 48,* 5–6. doi: 10.1111/j.1526-4610.2007.00968.x

Phillips, C., & Hunter, M. (1981). The treatment of tension headache: I. Muscular abnormality and biofeedback. *Behaviour Research and Therapy, 19,* 485–489. doi: 10.1016/0005-7967(81)90075-9

Pietrobon, D., & Striessnig, J. (2003). Neurobiology of migraine. *Nature Reviews Neuroscience, 4*, 386–398. doi: 10.1038/nrn1102

Poppen, P. (1987). *Behavioral relaxation training and assessment.* New York: Pergamon.

Powers, S. W., Kashikar-Zuck, S. M., Allen, J. R., LeCates, S. L., Slater, S. K., Zafar, M., … Hershey, A. D. (2013). Cognitive behavioral therapy plus amitriptyline for chronic migraine in children and adolescents: A randomized clinical trial. *Journal of the American Medical Association, 310*, 2622–2630. doi: 10.1001/jama.2013.282533

Powers, S. W., Mitchell, M. J., Byars, K. C., Bentti, A. L., LeCates, S. L., & Hersey, A. D. (2001). A pilot study of one-session biofeedback training in pediatric headache. *Neurology, 56*, 133. doi: 10.1212/WNL.56.1.133

Radat, F., Creac'h, C., Swendsen, J. D., Lafittau, M., Irachabal, S., Dousset, V., & Henry, P. (2005). Psychiatric comorbidity in the evolution from migraine to medication overuse headache. *Cephalalgia, 25*, 519–522. doi: 10.1111/j.1468-2982.2005.00910.x

Radat, F., & Swendsen, J. (2005). Psychiatric comorbidity in migraine: a review. *Cephalalgia, 25*, 165–178. doi: 10.1111/j.1468-2982.2004.00839.x

Rains, J. C., Lipchik, G. A., & Penzien, D. B. (2006). Behavioral facilitation of medical treatment for headache: Part I: Review of headache treatment compliance. *Headache, 46*, 1387–1394. doi: 10.1111/j.1526-4610.2006.00581.x

Rains, J. C., & Penzien, D. B. (2005). Behavioral research and the double-blind placebo-controlled methodology: Challenges in applying the biomedical standard to behavioral headache research. *Headache, 45*, 479–486. doi: 10.1111/j.1526-4610.2005.05099.x

Rains, J. C., Penzien, D. B., & Lipchik, G. A. (2006). Behavioral facilitation of medical treatment for headache: Part II: Theoretical models and behavioral strategies for improving adherence. *Headache, 46*, 1395–1403. doi: 10.1111/j.1526-4610.2006.00565.x

Rains, J. C., Penzien, D. B., McCrory, D. C., & Gray, R. N. (2005). Behavioral headache treatment: History, review of the empirical literature, and methodological critique. *Headache, 45*, S91–S108. doi: 10.1111/j.1526-4610.2005.4502003.x

Rains, J. C., & Poceta, J. S. (2006). Headache and sleep disorders: Review and clinical implications for headache management. *Headache, 46*, 1344–1363. doi: 10.1111/j.1526-4610.2006.00578.x

Robbins, L. (1994). Precipitating factors in migraine: A retrospective review of 494 patients. *Headache, 34*, 214–216

Rokicki, L. A., Holroyd, K. A., France, C. R., Lipchik, G. L., France, J. L., & Kvaal, S. A. (1997). Change mechanisms associated with combined relaxation/EMG biofeedback training for chronic tension headache. *Applied Psychophysiology and Biofeedback, 22*, 21–41.

Rothrock, J. F. (2008). The truth about triggers. *Headache, 3*, 499–500. doi: 10.1111/j.1526-4610.2007.01050.x

Rothrock, J. F., Parada, V. A., Sims, C., Key, K., Walters, N. S., & Zweifler, R. M. (2006). The impact of intensive patient education on clinical outcome in a clinic-based migraine population. *Headache, 46*, 726–731. doi: 10.1111/j.1526-4610.2006.00428.x

Rowan, A. B., & Andrasik, F. (1996). Efficacy and cost-effectiveness of minimal therapist contact treatments of chronic headache: A review. *Behavior Therapy, 27*, 207–234. doi: 10.1016/S0005-7894(96)80015-3

Saper, J. R., & Lake, A. E. (2002). Borderline personality disorder and the chronic headache patient: review and management recommendations. *Headache, 42*, 663–674. doi: 10.1046/j.1526-4610.2002.02156.x

Sarafino, E. P., & Goehring, B. A. (2000). Age comparisons in acquiring biofeedback control and success in reducing headache pain. *Annals of Behavioral Medicine, 22*, 10–16. doi: 10.1007/BF02895163

Sargent, J. D., Green, E. E., & Walters, E. D. (1972). The use of autogenic feedback training in a pilot study of migraine and tension headaches. *Headache, 12*, 120–124. doi: 10.1111/j.1526-4610.1972.hed1203120.x

Saunders, K., Merikangas, K., Low, N. C. P., Von Korff, M., & Kessler, R. C. (2008). Impact of comorbidity on headache-related disability. *Neurology, 70*, 534–547. doi: 10.1212/01.wnl.0000297192.84581.21

Schafer, A. M., Rains, J. C., Penzien, D. B., Groban, L., Smitherman, T. A., & Houle, T. T. (2011). Direct costs of preventive headache treatments: Comparison of behavioral and pharmacologic approaches. *Headache, 51,* 985–991. doi: 10.1111/j.1526-4610.2011.01905.x

Scharff, L., Turk, D. C., & Marcus, D.A. (1995). The relationship of locus of control and psychosocial-behavioral response in chronic headache. *Headache, 35,* 527–533. doi: 10.1111/j.1526-4610.1995.hed3509527.x

Scher, A. I., Stewart, W. F., Ricci, J. A., & Lipton, R. B. (2003). Factors associated with the onset and remission of chronic daily headache in a population-based study. *Pain, 106,* 81–89. doi: 10.1016/S0304-3959(03)00293-8

Scher, A. I., Midgette, L. A., & Lipton, R. B. (2008). Risk factors for headache chronification. *Headache, 48,* 16–25. doi: 10.1111/j.1526-4610.2007.00970.x

Schreiber, C. P., Hutchinson, S., Webster, C. J., Ames, M., Richardson, M. S., & Powers, C. (2004). Prevalence of migraine in patients with a history of self-reported or physician-diagnosed "sinus" headache. *Archives of Internal Medicine, 164,* 1769–1772. doi: 10.1001/archinte.164.16.1769

Schwartz, B. S., Stewart, W. F., Simon, D., & Lipton, R. B. (1998). Epidemiology of tension-type headache. *JAMA, 279,* 381–383. doi: 10.1001/jama.279.5.381

Schwartz, G. E., & Weiss, S. M. (1978). Behavioral medicine revisited: An amended definition. *Journal of Behavioral Medicine, 1,* 249–251. doi: 10.1007/BF00846677

Schwartz, M. S., & Andrasik, F. (Eds.). (2003). *Biofeedback: A practitioner's guide* (3rd ed.). New York, NY: Guilford.

Schürks, M., Rist, P. M., Bigal, M. E., Buring, J. E., Lipton, R. B., & Kurth, T. (2009). Migraine and cardiovascular disease: Systematic review and meta-analysis. *British Medical Journal, 339,* b3914. Retrieved from http://www.bmj.com/content/339/bmj.b3914.

Selye, H. A. (1936). A syndrome produced by diverse nocuous agents. *Nature, 138,* 32. doi: 10.1038/138032a0

Sempere, A. P., Porta-Etessam, J., Medrano, V., Garcia-Morales, I., Concepción, L., Ramos, A., . . . Botella, C. (2005). Neuroimaging in the evaluation of patients with non-acute headache. *Cephalalgia, 25,* 30–35. doi: 10.1111/j.1468-2982.2004.00798.x

Shapiro, D. & Schwartz, G. E. (1972). Biofeedback and visceral learning: Clinical applications. *Seminars in Psychiatry, 4,* 171–184.

Silberstein, S. D. (2000). Practice parameter: evidence-based guidelines for migraine headache (an evidence-based review): Report of the Quality Standards Subcommittee of the American Academy of Neurology. *Neurology, 55,* 754–762. doi: 10.1212/WNL.55.6.754

Silberstein, S. D., Holland, S., Freitag, F., Dodick, D. W., Argoff, C., & Ashman, E. (2012). Evidence-based guideline update: pharmacologic treatment for episodic migraine prevention in adults: Report of the Quality Standards Subcommittee of the American Academy of Neurology and the American Headache Society. *Neurology, 78,* 1337–1345. doi: 10.1212/WNL.0b013e3182535d20

Simmons, L. W., & Wolff, L. W. (1954). *Social science in medicine.* New York, NY: Russell Sage Foundation.

Smitherman, T. A., Burch, R., Sheikh, H., & Loder, E. (2013). The prevalence, impact and treatment of migraine and severe headaches in the United States: A review of statistics from national surveillance studies. *Headache, 53,* 427–436. doi: 10.1111/head.12074

Smitherman, T. A., & Kolivas, E. D. (2013). Trauma exposure versus posttraumatic stress disorder: Relative associations with migraine. *Headache, 53,* 775–786. doi: 10.1111/head.12063

Smitherman, T. A., Kolivas, E. D., & Bailey, J. R. (2013). Panic disorder and migraine: Comorbidity, mechanisms, and clinical implications. *Headache, 53,* 23–45. doi: 10.1111/head.12004

Smitherman, T. A., Maizels, M., & Penzien, D. B. (2008). Headache chronification: Screening and behavioral management of comorbid depressive and anxiety disorders. *Headache, 48,* 45–50. doi: 10.1111/j.1526-4610.2007.00974.x

Smitherman, T. A., Penzien, D. B., & Maizels, M. (2008). Anxiety disorders and migraine intractability and progression. *Current Pain and Headache Reports, 12,* 224–229. doi: 10.1007/s11916-008-0039-9

Smitherman, T. A., Rains, J. C., & Penzien, D. B. (2009). Psychiatric comorbidities and migraine chronification. *Current Pain and Headache Reports, 13*, 326–331. doi: 10.1007/s11916-009-0052-7

Smitherman, T. A., Walters, A. B., Maizels, M., & Penzien, D. B. (2011). The use of antidepressants for headache prophylaxis. *CNS Neuroscience & Therapeutics, 17*, 462–469. doi: 10.1111/j.1755-5949.2010.00170.x

Spitzer, R. L., Kroenke, K., Williams, J. B. W., & Löwe, B. (2006). A brief measure for assessing generalized anxiety disorder. *Archives of Internal Medicine, 166*, 1092–1097. doi: 10.1001/archinte.166.10.1092

Stewart, W. F., Lipton, R. B., Kolodner, K., Liberman, J., & Sawyer, J. (1999). Reliability of the Migraine Disability Assessment score in a population-based sample of headache sufferers. *Cephalalgia, 19*, 107–114. doi: 10.1046/j.1468-2982.1999.019002107.x

Stewart, W. F., Wood, C., Reed, M. L., Roy, J., & Lipton, R. B. (2008). Cumulative lifetime migraine incidence in women and men. *Cephalalgia, 28*, 1170–1178. doi: 10.1111/j.1468-2982.2008.01666.x

Stovner, L. J., Hagen, K., Jensen, R., Katsarava, Z., Lipton, R., Scher, A., ... Zwart, J.-A. (2007). The global burden of headache: A documentation of headache prevalence and disability worldwide. *Cephalalgia, 27*, 193–210. doi: 10.1111/j.1468-2982.2007.01288.x

Tietjen, G. E., & Peterlin, B. L. (2011). Childhood abuse and migraine: Epidemiology, sex differences, and potential mechanisms. *Headache, 51*, 869–879. doi: 10.1111/j.1526-4610.2011.01906.x

Trautmann, E., & Kröner-Herwig, B. (2010). A randomized controlled trial of Internet-based self-help training for recurrent headache in childhood and adolescence. *Behaviour Research and Therapy, 48*, 28–37. doi: 10.1016/j.brat.2009.09.004

Trautmann, E., Lackschewitz, H., & Kröner-Herwig, B. (2006). Psychological treatment of recurrent headache in children and adolescents: a meta-analysis. *Cephalalgia, 26*, 1411–1426. doi: 10.1111/j.1468-2982.2006.01226.x

Turner, D. P., & Houle, T. T. (2013). Psychological evaluation of a primary headache patient. *Pain Management, 3*, 19–25. doi: 10.2217/pmt.12.77

Turner, D. P., Smitherman, T. A., Martin, V., Penzien, D. B., & Houle, T. T. (2013). Causality and headache triggers. *Headache, 53*, 628–635. doi: 10.1111/head.12076

Vos, T., Flaxman, A. D., Naghavi, M., Lozano, R., Michaud, C., Exxati, M., ... Murray, C. J. L. (2012). Years lived with disability (YLDs) for 1160 sequelae of 289 diseases and injuries 1990–2010: A systematic analysis for the Global Burden of Disease Study 2010. *Lancet, 380*, 2163–2196. doi: 10.1016/S0140-6736(12)61729-2

Wessman, M., Terwindt, G. M., Kaunisto, M. A., Palotie, A., & Ophoff, R. A. (2007). Migraine: A complex genetic disorder. *Lancet Neurology, 6*, 521–532. doi: 10.1016/S1474-4422(07)70126-6

Wöber, C., Brannath, W., Schmidt, K., Kapitan, M., Rudel, E., Wessely, P., ... PAMINA Study Group. (2007). Prospective analysis of factors related to migraine attacks: the PAMINA study. *Cephalalgia, 27*, 304–314. doi: 10.1111/j.1468-2982.2007.01279.x

Wolff, H. (1948). *Headache and other head pain.* New York, NY: Oxford University Press.

8

Appendix: Tools and Resources

Detailed Headache Self-Monitoring Form

NAME:

PATIENT ID:

DIRECTIONS: Four times each day, please rate your headache intensity, disability level, and stress using the rating scales below. Mark the times that you were sleeping and eating by coloring (or putting an x) in the boxes. You may indicate ½ hour increments by coloring ½ of a box (or use a slash). Also, record body temperature, whether menstruating, and ratings of sleep amount and sleep quality.

HEADACHE INTENSITY

10 EXTREMELY PAINFUL . . My headache is so painful that I can't do anything.
9
8 VERY PAINFUL . . . . My headache makes concentration difficult, but I can perform demanding tasks.
7
6 PAINFUL. . . . . My headache is painful, but I can continue what I am doing.
5
4 MILDLY PAINFUL . . . . I can ignore my headache most of the time.
3
2 SLIGHTLY PAINFUL . . . . . I only notice my headache when I focus my attention on it.
1
0 NO HEADACHE

DISABILITY

10 COMPLETELY IMPAIRED (Bedrest)
9
8 SEVERELY IMPAIRED
7
6 MODERATELY IMPAIRED
5
4 MILDLY IMPAIRED
3
2 MINIMALLY IMPAIRED
1
0 NO IMPAIRMENT

STRESS

10 EXTREMELY
9
8 VERY
7
6 MODERATELY
5
4 MILDLY
3
2 SLIGHTLY
1
0 NO STRESS

SLEEP AMOUNT

10 TOO MUCH
9
8
7
6
5 PERFECT
4
3
2
1
0 TOO LITTLE

SLEEP QUALITY

10 EXCELLENT
9
8 VERY GOOD
7
6 GOOD
5
4 FAIR
3
2 POOR
1
0 VERY POOR

WEEKLY MEDICATION LIST (AND AMOUNT)

MONDAY	DATE:	12a	1a	2a	3a	4a	5a	6a	7a	8a	9a	10a	11a	12p	1p	2p	3p	4p	5p	6p	7p	8p	9p	10p	11p	
	HEADACHE																									TEMP
	DISABILITY																									MENSES Y – N
	STRESS																									SLEEP QUALITY
	SLEEP																									SLEEP QUALITY
	MEAL/SNACK																									

MEDICATION (AND AMOUNT)

COMMENTS:

TUESDAY

DATE: _____

	12a	1a	2a	3a	4a	5a	6a	7a	8a	9a	10a	11a	12p	1p	2p	3p	4p	5p	6p	7p	8p	9p	10p	11p	
HEADACHE																									TEMP
DISABILITY																									MENSES Y – N
STRESS																									SLEEP QUALITY
SLEEP																									SLEEP QUALITY
MEAL/SNACK																									
MEDICATION (AND AMOUNT)													COMMENTS:												

WEDNESDAY

DATE: _____

	12a	1a	2a	3a	4a	5a	6a	7a	8a	9a	10a	11a	12p	1p	2p	3p	4p	5p	6p	7p	8p	9p	10p	11p	
HEADACHE																									TEMP
DISABILITY																									MENSES Y – N
STRESS																									SLEEP QUALITY
SLEEP																									SLEEP QUALITY
MEAL/SNACK																									
MEDICATION (AND AMOUNT)													COMMENTS:												

THURSDAY

DATE: _____

	12a	1a	2a	3a	4a	5a	6a	7a	8a	9a	10a	11a	12p	1p	2p	3p	4p	5p	6p	7p	8p	9p	10p	11p	
HEADACHE																									TEMP
DISABILITY																									MENSES Y – N
STRESS																									SLEEP QUALITY
SLEEP																									SLEEP QUALITY
MEAL/SNACK																									
MEDICATION (AND AMOUNT)													COMMENTS:												

FRIDAY

DATE: _____

	12a	1a	2a	3a	4a	5a	6a	7a	8a	9a	10a	11a	12p	1p	2p	3p	4p	5p	6p	7p	8p	9p	10p	11p	
HEADACHE																									TEMP
DISABILTY																									MENSES Y – N
STRESS																									SLEEP QUALITY
SLEEP																									SLEEP QUALITY
MEAL/SNACK																									

MEDICATION (AND AMOUNT)

COMMENTS:

SATURDAY

DATE: _____

	12a	1a	2a	3a	4a	5a	6a	7a	8a	9a	10a	11a	12p	1p	2p	3p	4p	5p	6p	7p	8p	9p	10p	11p	
HEADACHE																									TEMP
DISABILTY																									MENSES Y – N
STRESS																									SLEEP QUALITY
SLEEP																									SLEEP QUALITY
MEAL/SNACK																									

MEDICATION (AND AMOUNT)

COMMENTS:

SUNDAY

DATE: _____

	12a	1a	2a	3a	4a	5a	6a	7a	8a	9a	10a	11a	12p	1p	2p	3p	4p	5p	6p	7p	8p	9p	10p	11p	
HEADACHE																									TEMP
DISABILTY																									MENSES Y – N
STRESS																									SLEEP QUALITY
SLEEP																									SLEEP QUALITY
MEAL/SNACK																									

MEDICATION (AND AMOUNT)

COMMENTS:

Brief Headache Self-Monitoring Form

Complete this BEFORE GOING TO BED each day

	Monday: __ /__ /__	Tuesday: __ /__ /__	Wednesday: __ /__ /__	Thursday: __ /__ /__	Friday: __ /__ /__	Saturday: __ /__ /__	Sunday: __ /__ /__
Did you have a headache today? (circle one)	Yes/No	Yes/No	Yes/No	Yes/No	Yes/No	Yes/No	Yes/No
If YES, how severe was the pain (0–10)?	____ (0–10)	____ (0–10)	____ (0–10)	____ (0–10)	____ (0–10)	____ (0–10)	____ (0–10)
If YES, how long did the headache last?	____ hours	____ hours	____ hours	____ hours	____ hours	____ hours	____ hours
If YES, What symptoms did you have with this headache? (check all that apply)	__ One-sided __ Throbbing __ Made worse by activity __ Nausea __ Vomiting __ Light sensitivity __ Sound sensitivity	__ One-sided __ Throbbing __ Made worse by activity __ Nausea __ Vomiting __ Light sensitivity __ Sound sensitivity	__ One-sided __ Throbbing __ Made worse by activity __ Nausea __ Vomiting __ Light sensitivity __ Sound sensitivity	__ One-sided __ Throbbing __ Made worse by activity __ Nausea __ Vomiting __ Light sensitivity __ Sound sensitivity	__ One-sided __ Throbbing __ Made worse by activity __ Nausea __ Vomiting __ Light sensitivity __ Sound sensitivity	__ One-sided __ Throbbing __ Made worse by activity __ Nausea __ Vomiting __ Light sensitivity __ Sound sensitivity	__ One-sided __ Throbbing __ Made worse by activity __ Nausea __ Vomiting __ Light sensitivity __ Sound sensitivity

Instructions for Detailed Headache Self-Monitoring

These forms are designed to help you keep a careful record of your: daily headache intensity levels, stress, disability, medication use, meal pattern, sleep (pattern, quality, amount), and menstruation (women only). Each page contains seven grids – one for each day of the week. You may want to fold the sheet so you can carry it with you in your pocket or purse. These boxes will be used to keep track of headache intensity, disability, stress, sleep, and meals/snacks. On top of the page are rating scales for headache intensity, disability, stress, sleep amount, and sleep quality. There are also boxes for keeping track of medications taken.

We would like you to rate each day's headache intensity, disability, and stress **AT LEAST TWICE** each day. Most people find it easiest to make their ratings around the same times each day. People also find it helpful to pair the act of recording with some other daily activity to help them remember to record. For example, you might record (1) at breakfast or when you first get up, (2) at lunch, and (3) at dinner or when you first get home from work or school. If you forget to make a recording at your usual time, please fill in the grid just as soon as you remember. In addition, whenever you take medication for a headache, please indicate the type and amount of medication in the space provided for that day.

Each time you update the grid put the ratings in the boxes that correspond to the time of day that you are rating. For example, if you are making ratings for 6 a.m. Monday, then indicate the level of your headache, disability, and stress in the boxes of the column for 6 a.m. Monday. Put the number in the box that best describes how you are feeling at that time. For headache intensity you will put a number from 0 (*NO HEADACHE*) to 10 (*EXTREMELY PAINFUL HEADACHE*), for disability level you will put a number from 0 (*NO IMPAIRMENT*) to 10 (*COMPLETELY IMPAIRED*), and for stress you will put a number from 0 (*NO STRESS*) to 10 (*EXTREMELY STRESSED*). Don't be overly concerned with the exact rating level you select; your first impression is probably the best estimate. If you have a day with no headache, please be sure to complete the grid anyway. To indicate your sleeping pattern, you will place an "X" in the boxes that correspond with times that you were asleep since your last rating. If you slept for only half of the hour, then place a "/" in the box. The boxes to the right side should be used to record your sleep amount and sleep quality based on your sleep from the previous night. For indicating meals and snacks, place an "X" in the hourly boxes that correspond with times of the day that you ate a meal or a snack.

Be sure to write your name and dates of the week on each page. **A sample of one's day monitoring is provided at the end of these instructions.** If you have any questions about the self-monitoring procedures, feel free to call and ask for advice.

From: T. A. Smitherman et al.: *Headache*   © 2015 Hogrefe Publishing

Detailed Headache Self-Monitoring Form (Sample)

NAME: *Betty Migraine*   PATIENT ID:

DIRECTIONS: Four times each day, please rate your headache intensity, disability level, and stress using the rating scales below. Mark the times that you were sleeping and eating by coloring (or putting an x) in the boxes. You may indicate ½ hour increments by coloring ½ of a box (or use a slash). Also, record body temperature, whether menstruating, and ratings of sleep amount and sleep quality.

HEADACHE INTENSITY

10 EXTREMELY PAINFUL .. My headache is so painful that I can't do anything.
9
8 VERY PAINFUL .... My headache makes concentration difficult, but I can perform demanding tasks.
7
6 PAINFUL.............. My headache is painful, but I can continue what I am doing.
5
4 MILDLY PAINFUL ...... I can ignore my headache most of the time.
3
2 SLIGHTLY PAINFUL .... I only notice my headache when I focus my attention on it.
1
0 NO HEADACHE

DISABILITY

10 COMPLETELY IMPAIRED (Bedrest)
9
8 SEVERELY IMPAIRED
7
6 MODERATELY IMPAIRED
5
4 MILDLY IMPAIRED
3
2 MINIMALLY IMPAIRED
1
0 NO IMPAIRMENT

STRESS

10 EXTREMELY
9
8 VERY
7
6 MODERATELY
5
4 MILDLY
3
2 SLIGHTLY
1
0 NO STRESS

SLEEP AMOUNT

10 TOO MUCH
9
8
7
6
5 PERFECT
4
3
2
1
0 TOO LITTLE

SLEEP QUALITY

10 EXCELLENT
9
8 VERY GOOD
7
6 GOOD
5
4 FAIR
3
2 POOR
1
0 VERY POOR

WEEKLY MEDICATION LIST (AND AMOUNT)

amitriptyline 50 mg at bedtime

MONDAY

DATE:	12a	1a	2a	3a	4a	5a	6a	7a	8a	9a	10a	11a	12p	1p	2p	3p	4p	5p	6p	7p	8p	9p	10p	11p
HEADACHE	0								0						7					4				
DISABILTY	0								0						7					4				
STRESS	4						6		6						8					6				
SLEEP		X	X	X	X	X	X																X	X
MEAL/SNACK									X					X		X				X				

MEDICATION (AND AMOUNT)

sumatriptan 100 mg at 2pm

COMMENTS: *left work with migraine*

	6p	7p	8p	9p	10p	11p	TEMP

MENSES
Y – (N)

SLEEP AMOUNT
3

SLEEP QUALITY
8

© 2015 Hogrefe Publishing

Structured Diagnostic Interview for Headache–3 (Brief Version)

Patient Name: _____ **Age:** _____ **Sex:** M   F

Patient ID: _____ **Interviewer:** _____ **Date:** / /

The following items are adapted from the Structured Diagnostic Interview for Headache (SDIH), part of the Headache Evaluation and Diagnostic System (HEDS), which includes software for data entry and diagnostic decision making. These materials are intended to facilitate diagnosis of selected recurrent, benign headaches according to ICHD-3 beta (2013) diagnostic criteria. Optimal use of this interview requires expertise with the diagnostic classification.

1. Does the patient get more than one type of headache? ☐ Yes ☐ No
   (If YES, complete a separate brief interview form for each type of headache) Headache #1 #2 #3

2. Select all pain locations that apply to this type of headache: *(You must check at least one)*

   ☐ frontal (A) ☐ temporal (B) ☐ occipital (C) ☐ orbital (D) ☐ supraorbital (E)

3. Select all that apply: ☐ top of head (F) ☐ base of neck (G) ☐ nasal/facial (H)

4. What is the intensity of pain that the patient experiences with a typical headache?
   _____ *(Indicate rating from 0–10)*

0	1	2	3	4	5	6	7	8	9	10
No Pain		Slightly Painful		Mildly Painful		Painful		Very Painful		Extremely Painful

---

5. Which of the following symptoms are a "predominant feature" of this headache type (presume that the headache is untreated)?

Pain location *(Select **only** one)*: ☐ Unilateral   ☐ Not unilateral

Pain features *(Select **only** one)*: ☐ Pulsating   ☐ Pressing/tightening (non-pulsating)

☐ Other: _____

6. How often does the patient experience this type of headache pain?

_____ w m y *(Indicate frequency in DAYS per **week**, **month**, or **year**; query headache-free days if patient has very frequent attacks or difficulty specifying days with headache)*

7. How long have these headaches been occurring at this rate?   _____ Months or _____ Years

8. What is the total number of this type of headache ever experienced:

☐ 1 ☐ 2–4 ☐ 5–9 ☐ >10 _____ *(Indicate total number experienced)*

9. How long does this headache last <u>if untreated or unsuccessfully treated</u>? (If patient falls asleep and wakes up without headache, duration of attack is until waking up. Check *unremitting* if patient reports never experiencing headache less than 7 days in duration). *(Indicate duration in **minutes**, **hours**, or **days**)*

_____ m h d Typical Average   _____ m h d Typical Minimum   _____ m h d Typical Maximum

OR ☐ Unremitting

10. Has anything about this headache (except frequency) changed in the last 6 months? ☐ Yes ☐ No

If **YES**, explain:

_____

_____

11. Is the patient's typical <u>headache pain</u> aggravated by (or cause avoidance of) routine physical activities (i.e., walking, climbing stairs, lifting, bending, etc.)?

☐ Yes ☐ No

12. Do any of the following symptoms occur with this headache?

☐ Headache worsened by conversational noise levels (phonophobia)
☐ Headache worsened by normal light (photophobia)
☐ Nausea *(Indicate intensity)*   ☐ Mild   ☐ Moderate   ☐ Severe
☐ Vomiting *(Indicate intensity)*   ☐ Mild   ☐ Moderate   ☐ Severe

13. Does the patient ever experience symptoms before this headache pain begins? ☐ Yes ☐ No

If **YES**, and if any of the reported symptoms provide evidence of visual, sensory, or other CNS symptoms, complete **Section 4a**

If **NO**, skip to #14

14. Does this headache have severe unilateral orbital, supraorbital, and/or temporal pain, and/or does the interviewer suspect a cluster-type headache? ☐ Yes ☐ No

If **YES**, complete **Section 4b**

If **NO**, skip to #15

From: T. A. Smitherman et al.: *Headache*

15. Does the patient use any medications to relieve headache pain? ☐ Yes ☐ No
    If **YES**, complete #15a, #15b
    If **NO**, skip to #16

    15a. How long has the patient been using the medication(s) to relieve headache pain?
        _____ d w m y *(Indicate in <u>d</u>ays, <u>w</u>eeks, <u>m</u>onths, or <u>y</u>ears)*

    15b. What is the frequency of medication use?
        _____ days per week _____ days per month _____ times per day
    If use has been occurring for >3 months and at a frequency of ≥ 2 days/week during this time, complete **Section 4c**
    If **NO**, skip to #16

16. Did this headache develop or worsen significantly (if pre-existing) after any trauma or injury to the head or neck? ☐ Yes ☐ No
    If **YES**, complete **Section 4d**
    If **NO**, skip to #17

17. Is this headache suspected to be attributed to another ICHD-3? ☐ Yes ☐ No
    17a. If aura symptoms are present, has transient ischemic attack been excluded? ☐ Yes ☐ No

---

Section 4a	**Migraine Aura Symptoms**

1. How many aura attacks has the patient experienced? _____

2. Which of the following apply to the aura symptoms? *(Select all that apply)*
    - ☐ At least one aura symptom spreads gradually over ≥ 5 minutes, **<u>AND/OR</u>** 2 or more symptoms occur in succession
    - ☐ Each individual aura symptom lasts 5–60 minutes
    - ☐ At least one aura symptom is unilateral
    - ☐ The aura is accompanied, or followed within 60 minutes, by headache

3. Indicate which of the following aura symptoms are present during this type of headache: *(Select all that apply)*

X	SYMPTOM	X	SYMPTOM
☐	Partial loss of sight (scotoma)	☐	Uncoordinated movements (ataxia)
☐	Scintillation	☐	Dizziness (vertigo)
☐	Blurred vision	☐	Ringing in ears (tinnitus)
☐	Fortification spectra (zig-zag lines)	☐	Decreased hearing acuity
☐	Double vision	☐	Decreased level of consciousness
☐	Tingling or numbness (paresthesias)	☐	Aphasia or unclassifiable speech
☐	Weakness (paresis)	☐	Poorly articulated speech (dysarthria)
☐	Other:	☐	Other:

From: T. A. Smitherman et al.: *Headache*

Section 4b — Cluster Headache Symptoms

1. Have the headaches occurred in cluster periods? ☐ Yes ☐ No
   If **YES**, complete #1a and #1b
   If **NO**, skip to #2

   1a. What is the total number of cluster periods experienced? _____

   1b. What is the duration of cluster periods? _____ d w m y *(Indicate duration in __days__, __weeks__, __months__, or __years__)*

2. Are the headaches separated by remission periods? ☐ Yes ☐ No
   If **YES**, complete #2a
   If **NO**, skip to #3

   2a. What is the duration of remission periods? _____ d w m y *(Indicate duration in __days__, __weeks__, __months, or years__)*

3. Indicate which of the following symptoms are present, as well as side affected, during this type of headache: *(Select all that apply)*

X	SYMPTOM	SIDE	X	SYMPTOM	SIDE
☐	Red eye (conjunctival injection)	R L	☐	Forehead and facial sweating	R L
☐	Tearing of the eye (lacrimation)	R L	☐	Forehead and facial flushing	R L
☐	Nasal congestion	R L	☐	Eyelid swelling (oedema)	R L
☐	Runny nose (rhinorrhoea)	R L	☐	Drooping eyelid (ptosis)	R L
☐	Pupillary constriction (miosis)	R L	☐	Sensation of fullness in the ear	R L
☐	Restlessness or agitation		☐	Other:	

Section 4c — Medication-Overuse Headache Symptoms

1. Has intake of ergotamine, triptans, or opioids occured on 10 or more days per month, for over 3 months
   ☐ Yes ☐ No
   If **YES**, indicate drug(s): ☐ ergotamine ☐ triptan ☐ opioid _____

2. Has the patient's intake of simple analgesics (eg, acetaminophen, acetylsalicylic acid, other NSAID), occurred on 15 or more days per month, for over 3 months? ☐ Yes ☐ No
   If **YES**, indicate drug: _____

3. Has the patient's intake of combination analgesics occurred on 2 or more days per week, for 10 or more days per month, for over 3 months? ☐ Yes ☐ No
   If **YES**, indicate drugs: _____

4. Has intake of any *combination* of ergotamine, triptans, simple analgesics, NSAIDs, and/or opioids occurred on 10 or more days per month, for over 3 months (without overuse of any single class alone)? ☐ Yes ☐ No
   If **YES**, indicate drug(s): _____

Section 4d   Posttraumatic Headache Symptoms

1. Did headache develop within 7 days after head trauma (or after regaining consciousness, or after regaining the ability to sense and report pain)? ☐ Yes ☐ No

2. Was there a loss of consciousness associated with head trauma? ☐ Yes ☐ No
   If **YES**, complete #2a
   If **NO**, skip to #3

   2a. What was the duration of unconsciousness? _____ m h d *(Indicate duration in <u>m</u>inutes, <u>h</u>ours, or <u>d</u>ays)*

3. How long has the headache continued? *(Select most representative category)*
   ☐ Resolves within 3 months after head trauma
   ☐ Persists for greater than 3 months after head trauma
   ☐ Persists but 3 months have not passed since head trauma

4. Is head injury attributed to whiplash? ☐ Yes ☐ No
   If **YES**, skip #5 through #9
   If **NO**, complete #5 through #9

5. Did coma develop? ☐ Yes ☐ No
   If **YES**, indicate severity on Glasgow Coma Scale (GCS):
   ☐ GCS <13 *[moderate/severe]*   ☐ GCS >13 *[mild]*

6. Did post-traumatic amnesia develop and continue for longer than 24 hours? ☐ Yes ☐ No

7. Was there alteration in level of awareness for longer than 24 hours? ☐ Yes ☐ No

8. Were abnormal neuroimaging results attained suggestive of a traumatic head injury?
   ☐ Yes ☐ No

9. Immediately after the head injury, were any of the following present? *(Select all that apply)*
   ☐ Transient confusion, disorientation, or impaired consciousness
   ☐ Loss of memory for events immediately before or after the head injury
   ☐ At least two symptoms suggestive of mild traumatic brain injury (nausea, vomiting, visual disturbances, dizziness and/or vertigo, impaired memory and/or concentration) *(Circle all symptoms that apply)*

Structured Diagnostic Interview for Headache–3: Coding Checklist

Y	N		Migraine without aura
☐	☐	A.	Has the patient had at least five attacks fulfilling criteria B–D? **(Question #8 on SDIH-3)**
☐	☐	B.	Do the headache attacks last 4–72 hours (untreated or unsuccessfully treated)? **(#9)**
☐	☐	C.	Has the patient had at least two of the following characteristics? ☐ Unilateral location **(#5)** ☐ Pulsating quality **(#5)** ☐ Moderate or severe pain intensity **(#4)** ☐ Aggravation by or causing avoidance of routine physical activity **(#11)**
☐	☐	D.	Has the patient experienced at least 1 of the following during headache? **(#12)** ☐ Nausea and/or vomiting ☐ Photophobia AND phonophobia
☐	☐	E.	Is this headache attributed to another ICHD-3 disorder? **(#17)**
Y	**N**		**Migraine with aura**
			(Refer to Appendix 4, Section 4a)
☐	☐	A.	Has patient had at least two aura attacks fulfilling criterion B? **(Section 4a: #1)**
☐	☐	B.	Has the patient experienced aura consisting of at least one of the following fully reversible aura symptoms? **(Section 4a: #3)** ☐ Visual ☐ Sensory ☐ Speech/language ☐ Motor ☐ Brainstem ☐ Retinal
☐	☐	C.	Has patient had at least two of the following characteristics? **(Section 4a: #2)** ☐ At least one aura symptom spreads gradually over ≥ 5 minutes, and/or two or more symptoms occur in succession ☐ Each individual aura symptom lasts 5–60 minutes ☐ At least one aura symptom is unilateral ☐ The aura is accompanied, or followed within 60 minutes, by headache
☐	☐	D.	Is this headache attributed to another ICDH-3 disorder, and has transient ischemic attack been excluded? **(#17, #17a)**
Y	**N**		**Chronic migraine**
☐	☐	A.	Does patient experience headache (migraine-like or tension-type-like) on ≥ 15 or more days per month for > 3 months? **(#6, #7)**
☐	☐	B.	Has patient had at least 5 attacks fulfilling either criteria B–D for *Migraine without aura and/or criteria B and C for Migraine with aura*? **(See previous checklist sections)**

Y	N		
☐	☐	C.	On ≥ 8 days per month for > 3 months, does patient meet any of the following? (**#6, #7, #8, and previous checklist sections**) ☐ Criteria C and D for *Migraine without aura* ☐ Criteria B and C for *Migraine with aura* ☐ Attacks believed by the patient to be migraine at onset and relieved by a triptan or ergot derivative (**Query patient if needed**)
☐	☐	D.	Is this headache better accounted for by another ICHD-3 diagnosis? (**#17**)

Y	N		Tension-type headache (episodic and chronic)
☐	☐	A.	Does this headache last from 30 minutes to 7 days? (**#9**) (NOTE: headache can be *unremitting* in chronic TTH only)
☐	☐	B.	Does headache have at least two of the following characteristics? ☐ Bilateral location (**#5**) ☐ Pressing/tightening (nonpulsating) quality (**#5**) ☐ Mild or moderate pain intensity (**#4**) ☐ Not aggravated by routine physical activity such as walking, climbing stairs (**#11**)
☐	☐	C.	Does the patient experience BOTH of the following? (**#12**) ☐ No nausea and/or vomiting (NOTE: *mild* nausea can be present in chronic TTH only) ☐ No more than one of photophobia or phonophobia
☐	☐	D.	Is this headache a better accounted for by another ICHD-3 diagnosis? (**#17**)

			If the patient meets criteria for TTH, determine frequency:
☐	☐		Has the patient had at least 10 episodes occurring on < 1 day per month on average (< 12 days per year)? *[infrequent episodic]* (**#6, #8**)
☐	☐		Has the patient had at least 10 episodes occurring on > 1 but < 15 days per month on average for > 3 months (≥ 12 and < 180 days per year)? *[frequent episodic]* (**#6, #7, #8**)
☐	☐		Has the patient had headache on ≥15 days per month on average for > 3 months (≥ 180 days per year)? *[chronic]* (**#6, #7, #8**)

Y	N		Cluster headache
			(Refer to Appendix 4, Section 4b)
☐	☐	A.	Has patient experienced at least five attacks fulfilling criteria B–D? (**#8**)
☐	☐	B.	Does the patient experience severe or very severe unilateral orbital, supraorbital, and/or temporal pain lasting 15-180 min if untreated? (**#9, #14**)
☐	☐	C.	Is the headache accompanied by at least one of the following? (**Section 4b: #3**) ☐ Ipsilateral conjunctival injection and/or lacrimation ☐ Ipsilateral nasal congestion and/or rhinorrhea ☐ Ipsilateral eyelid edema ☐ Ipsilateral forehead and facial sweating ☐ Ipsilateral forehead and facial flushing ☐ Ipsilateral sensation of fullness in the ear ☐ Ipsilateral miosis and/or ptosis ☐ A sense of restlessness or agitation
☐	☐	D.	Do the headache attacks have a frequency from one every other day to eight per day when the disorder is active? (**#6; query patient if needed**)
☐	☐	E.	Is headache better accounted for by another ICHD-3 diagnosis? (**#17**)

From: T. A. Smitherman et al.: *Headache*

Y	N		
			If the patient meets criteria for cluster headache, determine chronicity:
☐	☐		Has the patient had at least two cluster periods lasting 7–365 days (when untreated) and separated by pain-free remission periods of ≥ 1 month? *[episodic]* **(Section 4b: #1, #1a, #1b, #2, #2a)**
☐	☐		Has the patient had attacks recur for at least 1 year without remission periods **OR** with remission periods lasting <1 month? *[chronic]* **(#7, Section 4b: #1, #2, #2a)**
Y	**N**		**Medication-overuse headache**
			(Refer to Appendix 4, Section 4c)
☐	☐		Has the headache occurred on ≥ 15 days per month? **(#6)**
☐	☐		Has there been regular overuse for greater than 3 months of one or more drugs? **(#15a, #15b)**
			If patient meets criteria for MOH, determine type of drug intake:
☐	☐		Has the patient's intake of ergotamine occurred on ≥ 10 days per month on a regular basis for > 3 months? *[ergotamine-overuse headache]* **(Section 4c: #1)**
☐	☐		Has the patient's intake of triptans occurred on ≥ 10 days per month on a regular basis for > 3 months? *[triptan-overuse headache]* **(Section 4c: #1)**
☐	☐		Has the patient's intake of opioids occurred on ≥10 days per month on a regular basis for >3 months? *[opioid-overuse headache]* **(Section 4c: #1)**
☐	☐		Has the patient's intake of simple analgesics/NSAIDs occurred on ≥ 15 days per month on a regular basis for > 3 months? *[simple analgesic-overuse headache]* **Section 4c: #2)**
☐	☐		Has the patient's intake of combination analgesics occurred on ≥ 10 days per month on a regular basis for > 3 months? *[combination analgesic-overuse headache]* **(Section 4c: #3)**
☐	☐		Has the patient's intake of any combination of ergotamine, triptans, analgesics, and/or opioids occurred on ≥ 10 days per month on a regular basis for > 3 months, without overuse of any single drug class? *[medication-overuse headache attributed to multiple drug classes not individually overused]* **(Section 4c: #4)**
Y	**N**		**Posttraumatic headache attributed to moderate or severe head injury**
			(Refer to Appendix 4, Section 4d)
☐	☐		Has the patient experienced a head trauma with at least one of the following? ☐ Loss of consciousness for > 30 min **(Section 4d: #2, #2a)** ☐ Glasgow Coma Scale < 13 **(Section 4d: #5)** ☐ Posttraumatic amnesia for > 24 hr **(Section 4d: #6)** ☐ Alteration in level of awareness for > 24 hours **(Section 4d: #7)** ☐ Imaging demonstration of a traumatic head injury (intracranial hemorrhage, brain contusion, etc.) **(Section 4d: #8)**
☐	☐		Did headache develop within 7 days after head trauma or after regaining consciousness following head trauma (or after regaining the ability to sense and report pain)? **(Section 4d: #1)**

			If patient meets criteria for moderate or severe PTHA, determine chronicity:

☐	☐		Has the patient experienced either of the following? *[acute]* (Section 4d: #3)
			  ☐ Headache resolves within 3 months after head trauma
			  ☐ Headache persists but 3 months have not yet passed since head trauma

☐	☐		Has the headache persisted for >3 months after head trauma? *[persistent]* (Section 4d: #3)
Y	**N**		**Posttraumatic headache attributed to mild head injury**
			(Refer to Appendix 4, Section 4d)

☐	☐		Has the patient experienced a head trauma meeting **ALL** of the following criteria?
			  ☐ Either no loss of consciousness, or loss of consciousness for < 30 min duration **(Section 4d: #2, #2a)**
			  ☐ Glasgow Coma Scale > 13 **(Section 4d: #5)**
			  ☐ Either no posttraumatic amnesia, or posttraumatic amnesia for ≤ 24 hours **(Section 4d: #6)**
			  ☐ Either no alteration in awareness, or alteration in awareness for ≤ 24 hours **(Section 4d: #7)**
			  ☐ No imaging findings suggestive of a traumatic head injury **(Section 4d: #8)**

☐	☐		Immediately following the head injury, were one or more of the following present? **(Section 4d: #9)**
			  ☐ Transient confusion, disorientation, or impaired consciousness
			  ☐ Loss of memory for events immediately before or after the head injury
			  ☐ At least two symptoms suggestive of mild traumatic brain injury (nausea, vomiting, visual disturbances, dizziness and/or vertigo, impaired memory and/or concentration)

☐	☐		Did the headache develop within 7 days after head trauma? **(Section 4d: #1)**
			If patient meets criteria for mild PTHA, determine chronicity:

☐	☐		Has the patient experienced either one or other of the following? *[acute]* (Section 4d: #3)
			  ☐ Headache resolves within 3 months after head trauma
			  ☐ Headache persists but 3 months have not yet passed since head trauma

☐	☐		Has the headache persisted for > 3 months after head trauma? *[persistent]* (Section 4d: #3)
Y	**N**		**Headache attributed to whiplash injury**
			(Refer to Appendix 4, Section 4d)
☐	☐		Has the patient experienced a history of whiplash associated at the time with neck pain and/or headache? **(Section 4d: #4)**
☐	☐		Did the headache develop within 7 days after whiplash injury? **(Section 4d: #1)**
			If patient meets criteria for mild PTHA attributed to whiplash, determine chronicity:

☐	☐		Has the patient experienced 1 either of the following? *[acute]* (Section 4d: #3)
			  ☐ Headache resolves within 3 months after whiplash injury
			  ☐ Headache persists but 3 months have not yet passed since whiplash injury

☐	☐		Has the headache persisted for > 3 months after whiplash injury? *[persistent]* (Section 4d: #3)

Relaxation Practice Log

Relaxation rating scale

| 0 | 1 | 2 | 3 | 4 | 5 | 6 | 7 | 8 | 9 | 10 |

Not at all relaxed   Extremely relaxed

		Beginning relaxation rating	End relaxation rating	Total practice time	Comments
Day 1 Date:	Practice 1				
	Practice 2				
	Practice 3				
Day 2 Date:	Practice 1				
	Practice 2				
	Practice 3				
Day 3 Date:	Practice 1				
	Practice 2				
	Practice 3				
Day 4 Date:	Practice 1				
	Practice 2				
	Practice 3				
Day 5 Date:	Practice 1				
	Practice 2				
	Practice 3				
Day 6 Date:	Practice 1				
	Practice 2				
	Practice 3				
Day 7 Date:	Practice 1				
	Practice 2				
	Practice 3				

From: T. A. Smitherman et al.: *Headache*   © 2015 Hogrefe Publishing

Thermal Biofeedback Practice Log

Relaxation rating scale

0	1	2	3	4	5	6	7	8	9	10
Not at all relaxed										Extremely relaxed

		Beginning Hand Temp	End Hand Temp	Beginning relaxation rating	End relaxation rating	Total practice time	Comments
Day 1 Date:	Practice 1						
	Practice 2						
	Practice 3						
Day 2 Date:	Practice 1						
	Practice 2						
	Practice 3						
Day 3 Date:	Practice 1						
	Practice 2						
	Practice 3						
Day 4 Date:	Practice 1						
	Practice 2						
	Practice 3						
Day 5 Date:	Practice 1						
	Practice 2						
	Practice 3						
Day 6 Date:	Practice 1						
	Practice 2						
	Practice 3						
Day 7 Date:	Practice 1						
	Practice 2						
	Practice 3						

From: T. A. Smitherman et al.: *Headache*
© 2015 Hogrefe Publishing

Stressful Situations Monitoring Form

	Situation (Describe the situation: what was happening, where it took place, who else was there)	Behaviors/thoughts/feelings (What were you doing, thinking, and feeling? Include at least 1 behavior, 1 thought, and 1 feeling)	Result (What was the outcome? How did you feel about it?)
Situation 1 Date: Day: Time: Headache? Y N			
Situation 2 Date: Day: Time: Headache? Y N			
Situation 3 Date: Day: Time: Headache? Y N			

From: T. A. Smitherman et al.: *Headache*

SOLVE Problems Worksheet

Problem rating scale

0	1	2	3	4	5	6	7	8	9	10
Not at all a problem										Very much a problem

1. **S**tate the problem:

   Problem rating _____

2. **O**utline the problem:

3. **L**ist possible solutions:	4. **V**iew the consequences:
(a)	+
	−
(b)	+
	−
(c)	+
	−
(d)	+
	−
(e)	+
	−
(f)	+
	−
5. **E**xecute your solution. Problem Rating _____	

From: T. A. Smitherman et al.: *Headache*
© 2015 Hogrefe Publishing

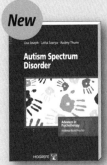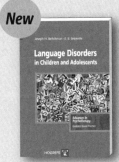
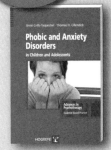
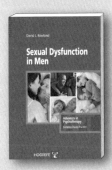
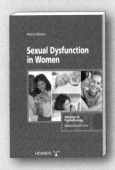
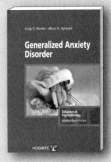
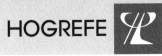

View all volumes at www.hogrefe.com/series/apt

Hogrefe Publishing
30 Amberwood Parkway · Ashland, OH 44805 · USA
Tel: (800) 228-3749 · Fax: (419) 281-6883
E-Mail: customerservice@hogrefe.com

Hogrefe Publishing
Merkelstr. 3 · 37085 Göttingen · Germany
Tel: +49 551 999 500 · Fax: +49 551 999 50 111
E-Mail: customerservice@hogrefe.de

Hogrefe Publishing c/o Marston Book Services Ltd
160 Eastern Ave., Milton Park · Abingdon, OX14 4SB · UK
Tel: +44 1235 465577 · Fax +44 1235 465556
direct.orders@marston.co.uk

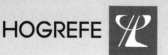

HOGREFE

Order online at **www.hogrefe.com**
or call toll-free **(800) 228-3749** (US only)